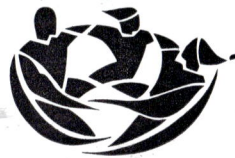

GW01374380

N AND MUSEUM SERVICES

NTRE,

THIS IS DUE BACK ON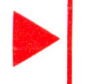

IT WAS LAST RETURNED ON

How to resolve the motherhood/career dilemma and have it all

SALE STOCK

PRICE: 10p

DATE:

03090647

TELEPEN

Double income, no kids . . . yet?

How to resolve the motherhood/career dilemma and have it all

MAUREEN MILLER

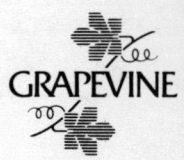

First published 1989

© Maureen Miller 1989

All rights reserved. No part of this book may be reproduced or utilized in any form or by any means, electronic or mechanical, including photocopying, recording or by any information storage and retrieval system, without permission in writing from the Publisher.

British Library Cataloguing in Publication Data

Miller, Maureen
  Double income, no kids — yet?
  1. Women. Pregnancy & childbirth — Manuals —
  For parents
  I. Title
  306.8'743

ISBN 0-7225-1736-X

Grapevine is part of the Thorsons Publishing Group, Wellingborough, Northamptonshire NN8 2RQ, England.

Typeset by Harper Phototypesetters Limited, Northampton
Printed and bound in Great Britain by Biddles Limited, Guildford, Surrey

10 9 8 7 6 5 4 3 2 1

Contents

	Introduction	7
CHAPTER ONE:	Are you going to have a family?	9
CHAPTER TWO:	When is the best time to have a baby?	17
CHAPTER THREE:	Coping with motherhood	29
CHAPTER FOUR:	Child-care and the working mother	38
CHAPTER FIVE:	Women and employment	51
CHAPTER SIX:	Finance and a family	71
CHAPTER SEVEN:	A word on behalf of fathers	78
	References and further information	84
	Index	93

Introduction

Deciding to have a baby is probably the most important decision any woman will ever make. By becoming a mother, a woman forfeits for ever her right to be single-minded and selfish about her life.

If you are one of the so-called new breed of high-flying executive woman, the question of when is the best time to have a baby is perhaps even more crucial for you, because it will bring you to a crossroads in your life at which you will have to choose between children and a career, or take the bold decision to combine both.

This book examines some of the dilemmas involved in making this decision, and considers the impact having a baby might have on double-income, twin career couples.

It would be wrong to suggest that there is a single solution or a simple answer. Each couple must reach their decision on the basis of their lifestyle, career and income pressures. However, this book will help you focus on some of the key issues you will need to face up to when deciding whether or not to have a baby.

CHAPTER ONE
Are you going to have a family?

> *She took a look at life, for she had a clear sense of it there, something real, something private, which she shared neither with her children nor with her husband.*
> (Mrs Ramsay, *To The Lighthouse*, Virginia Woolf.)

'Are you going to have a family?' How many times have you been asked this question, sometimes even by complete strangers? They would not dream of asking you about your marital intentions, yet, time and time again, young working women are quizzed about their attitude towards motherhood and children. And, as if the question itself were not presumptuous enough, your answer will be further analysed. If your standard, polite reply goes something like, 'Yes, probably, at some stage', you will be asked whether you intend to carry on working; how many children you plan to have; how your husband or partner feels about the idea; how you feel about someone else looking after your child every day; and, anyway, aren't you more interested in your work than in having a baby?

What lies behind this endless fascination with a woman's maternal intentions are, perhaps, the more fundamental questions: What sort of woman are you? Do you plan to be a traditional wife and mother? Is your career more important to you than a husband and children? Do you intend to try to combine the two ideals of perfect devoted mother and high-flying career woman? – in fact, the very questions you should be asking yourself if you have reached that stage in your life when your biological clock has started ringing alarm bells.

If you are one of the so-called new breed of executive, high-flying woman, approaching the milestone ages of 30 or 40, or, if you are just starting out on a career, the question of how to combine motherhood with a career and your professional life might well be troubling you.

When is the best time to have a first baby? Am I already too old? Would this mean an extended career break? Would it be better to change my job and, perhaps, work part-time or freelance? Could we afford to do without my salary? How would I feel about going back to work? Who would I get to look after the baby? These are some of the questions you may be pondering if you are entering that phase in your life when maternal instinct is starting to compete with ambition for your undivided attention, and you are faced with the fundamental problem of how to combine having a child with the pressures of a full-time, demanding career.

But perhaps the most important question to ask yourself is what kind of woman you want to be. Do you feel that fulfilment as a wife and full-time mother is what you seek, or do you need the satisfaction and stimulation of having an independent life outside the home? Face up honestly to what sort of lifestyle you and your partner would like to have before you decide to have children. It would be grossly misleading to say that having a baby will not change your life, especially if you have waited a long time before becoming parents. It will have a profound impact on every aspect of your life. You will be disillusioned if you start out with a 'nothing will change' philosophy.

Of course, you could indulge your parental inclinations electronically. An American video company has come up with a product designed to give you 'enjoyment without commitment'. At the end of a hard day at the office, their film *Video Baby*, will allow you 13 blissful minutes of cooing at your 'screen' offspring, without the problem of sleepless nights and midnight feeds. If, however, such second-hand experience is not for you, you might like to consider some of the issues that will need to be resolved by you and your partner as you try to reconcile your desire to become a mother with a lifestyle, income and career aspirations you have grown accustomed to, perhaps for quite a number of years.

There can be no doubt that the conflict between career and children, ambition and maternal instinct, is probably the most significant dilemma in the life of many women and couples, especially if the woman has demonstrated her potential and success as a high achiever and a high income earner. Being a mother can seriously damage your earnings potential and disrupt your career path.

But what about so-called equal opportunities? How are women responding to the changing climate for women in business and industry, and what impact is this having on their decision to become mothers? If we look at current trends, we find that the evidence of research accumulated over a number of years points to the detrimental impact of childbearing in shaping and influencing women's employment experience and their earnings. Having children can cost a woman up to *half* her potential lifetime's earnings, with the two most critical factors being an inability to return to her original position on the career ladder, either with her old firm or a new company, and difficulties in finding acceptable child-care. Indeed, child-care has become an important issue throughout the European Community, particularly in the UK, which has the lowest employment rates for mothers of children under five.

However, despite all the obstacles in their way, many women are leaving behind the stereotypes of wife and mother or ruthlessly ambitious career woman. Marriages are being postponed until later in life, couples are tending to live together, women are opting for fewer children and having them in a shorter space of time, and either marking time in their career or returning to work as soon as they possibly can after the birth.

A couple of decades ago, if they had worked at all, women automatically gave up their jobs in order to get married, whether their husbands were company directors or factory workers. Whatever their husband's income, all women were equally dependent on their husband for financial support

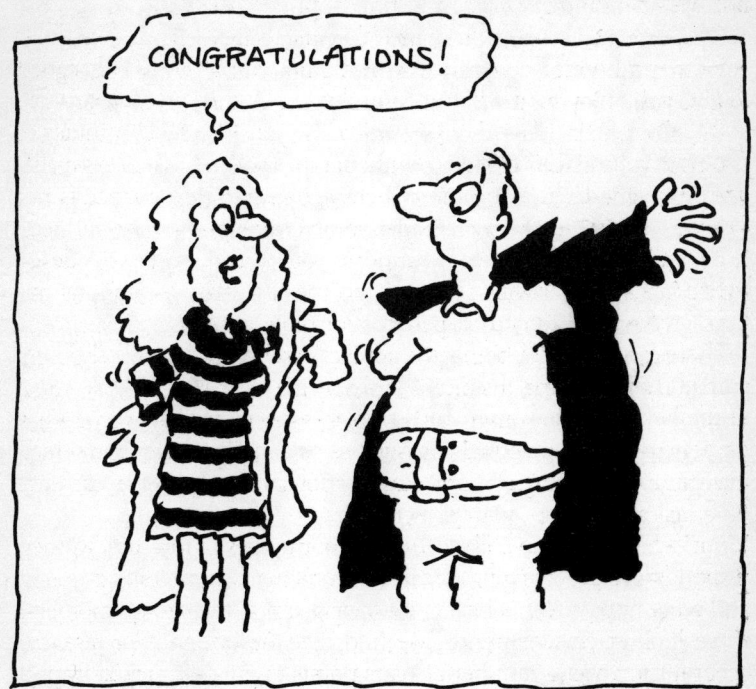

and personal fulfilment. But women today are not so homogeneous a group. The lure of financial independence and career fulfilment means that most women leave home and work full-time before they get married and continue to do so after their wedding. This trend has been so strong that women now make up over half the nation's workforce.

But these trends are changing, and we are witnessing the gradual breakdown of the 'traditional' pattern of family structure.

Indeed, only 8 per cent of British couples live in what advertisers would have us believe is the traditional marriage, with the wife staying at home to look after the children, while the husband goes out to work as the sole breadwinner.

The traditional role and lifestyle of many women has changed dramatically over the past decade. Now, most women return to work as soon as they practically can after the birth of their first baby, usually within the first year.

A major review of the changing role of women has predicted that women in Britain are ready to scramble free from their domestic mould and emerge as a vibrant new breed of independent, capable, high achievers and, more importantly, high earners. And, says the report, women regard work as crucial to their new-found independence, with more than half regarding motherhood as an interruption to their careers rather than as their main purpose in life. These changes have already begun to happen, and, although the majority of working women are in low-paid jobs in secretarial, shop and health sectors, the numbers of women entering the professions has doubled in the last ten years and continues to rise.

In spite of the broad recognition of these trends by society and industry, today's generation of working mothers are very much pioneers of the dual-income, dual-role lifestyle. It is true that many women have made it to the boardroom, and to the highest levels of professional life and feature among the country's most successful and imaginative entrepreneurs. They have also demonstrated that it *is* possible to combine ambition and ability with the role of wife and mother, and research indicates that in the next decade, women will consolidate their independence and compete with men for top positions in all areas of business and professional life. But these women who have gone down *both* the parallel routes of mother and career woman have only been able to achieve these twin goals through granite-like determination and sheer hard work. For, although women are becoming more integrated into senior positions in business and industry, the support systems to enable women to realize their potential at work are seriously inadequate.

Equal opportunity lobbyists are arguing that, in the 1990s, child-care will be the most sought-after perk. Until then, the double-income lifestyle effectively means double lives for those women who try to seek dual fulfilment in motherhood and a career.

Although equal opportunities in education, job openings and training are enabling women to achieve very real success in their working lives, this new generation of woman now finds herself isolated and unprepared for motherhood.

Indeed, many successful working women suffer from stereotyping as 'career women' as much as their full-time housewife and mother counterparts suffer from the derogatory label of 'just a housewife'. Very often, they find they are excluded from 'baby-talk' by full-time mothers, who assume that they are not interested, or will not understand. So, unless they can find a friend or colleague who has managed to combine the two roles, they may feel increasingly isolated and anxious as they try to work out their own response to the motherhood-career dilemma.

Motherhood is a strange, almost mystical state. In spite of the revolution in attitudes towards women, the image of a young, beautiful Madonna-like girl cradling a perfect, contented baby still clouds society's vision of motherhood. For many people, the highly competitive, successful career woman, competing on equal terms with men in an essentially male environment is tinged with a hint of the cold and the unnatural.

The maternal instinct is at its most mystical in the way in which it can strike you when you are least expecting it, just when you thought your priorities were firmly centred somewhere between your desk and your bank balance. A number of things can trigger off this emotional reaction: the sudden realization that, after ten or more years battling your way up the career ladder, although financially and materially rewarding, this single-minded approach to life is basically hollow and empty. A close friend or member of the family having a baby will very often unleash your own maternal instinct which you thought you had under control. Indeed, many career women are surprised by the overwhelming strength of the desire to have a baby when it finally strikes them. Having insisted for years that children were 'not for you', you will find your emotions at war with your rational attitudes to your work. Actually admitting to yourself that you *are* prepared to succumb to your own natural instinct is the first hurdle. If you have spent years projecting an image of a cool, hard-headed working-woman, you may feel that you are, in some way, betraying yourself by giving in to the most natural of female emotions.

For some, it will be an act of heroism to inform your employer and colleagues that you are pregnant.

The pressure of advancing years — the 'now or never' factor — may also bring the subject of having children to a head. For some successful, independent women, age is an important determinant, since the milestone of her thirtieth birthday may sharpen her realization that, having spent the past ten years concentrating on her job, her personal life has been neglected and she has not yet even found a man with whom she wants to share her life, let alone decided whether or not she wants children. Financially secure, it is very likely that she owns her home and logically she could support a child as a single parent, but what of the reactions of her family, society?

Pressure from your husband/partner and from your parents, longing for a first grandchild, is also a significant factor. This sort of pressure can be particularly difficult to resist, especially if you are a newly wed 20- or 25-year-old who wants to spend a few years establishing your track record at work before dealing with the issue of childbearing and motherhood. Bear in mind that, no matter how well meaning your husband may be about insisting that he will take a full part in looking

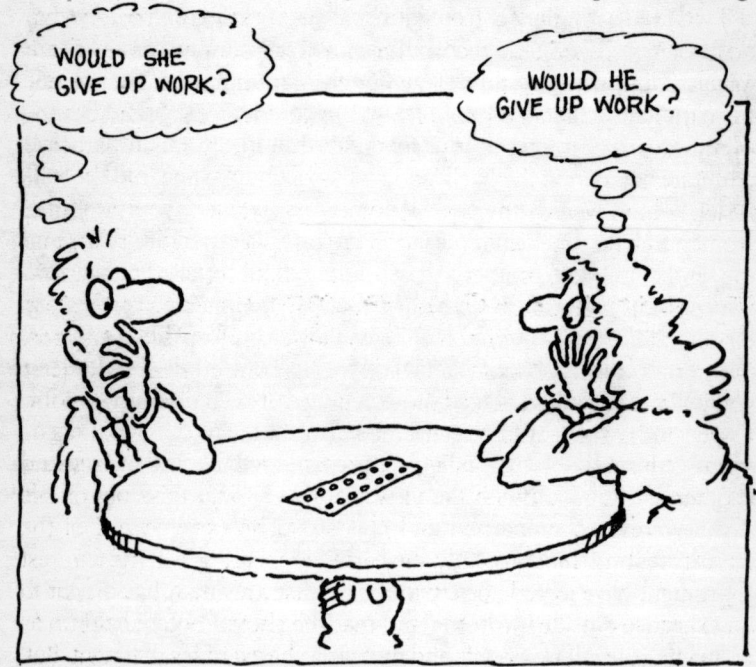

after the child, by far the greater share of that responsibility will actually fall to you. You must be sure that you are ready for that level of responsibility and commitment, whether you decide to become a full-time or a working mother, to prevent friction in your relationship with your husband once you have the child. This can be further complicated if the wife is in a job earning a higher salary with better career prospects than her husband, which is by no means uncommon. For such women to give up their job to have a baby is a greater financial sacrifice for the whole family's future quality of life.

An additional complication for some couples is the way in which marriage seems to be going out of fashion. Fewer couples marry now than did in the Sixties and early Seventies. The boom in women's jobs has been signalled as the most important reason why women no longer rush into marriage as a way of winning independence from their parents. For these couples, the decision to have a baby has to be considered alongside the other fundamental questions: whether they want to turn their partnership into a more legally binding, long-term commitment symbolized by marriage; and the moral and legal implications of having a child out of wedlock.

If your husband already has children from an earlier marriage, he may be fiercely opposed to repeating the experience simply to satisfy your maternal urges. This could be for a number of reasons, not least among them the financial implications of the possible loss of your salary, bearing in mind the heavy cost of supporting his first family. Much harder to admit to, however, is the likely fear he has of you turning into the wife he left behind, and that the well-groomed, confident, successful career woman to whom he was attracted in the first place may well turn into the kind of full-time mother and wife with whom he failed to maintain a successful and lasting relationship. You may find that the price to pay for this brand of motherhood is having to return to work afterwards. Only you can decide if you can abide by this compromise, but at least you will not have been denied the experience of having your own baby, whatever the subsequent arrangements.

For generations, young girls were prepared for the role of wife and mother and grew up with the view that they would miss out on life if they remained unmarried and childless. The extreme zeal of the suffragettes and, more recently, the fierce independence of the feminist movement have forced society to accept that a woman has a right to an existence outside the home, and that she should not be held up as an inadequate and poor wife and mother if she exercises that right. But, ironically, this new-found independence and freedom poses a heavy burden of choice on those women who feel drawn to both ways of life.

The important thing is to be honest about your ideals and goals. Everyone believes they are an expert on parenthood and children. Advice, most of it conflicting, will be heaped on you from all sides. It is important not to be pressurized about this, the most important of all the decisions you will ever make. Trust your instincts and have courage in your decision. Many women in all kinds of careers and domestic circumstances have found that it is possible to combine a career with being a mother. Whatever you decide, it is a decision and a way of life that will be with you for a very long time.

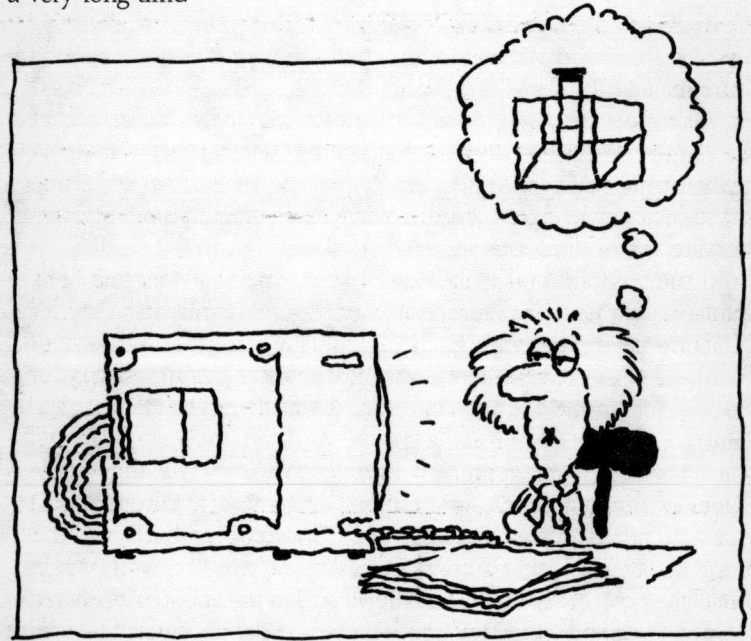

CHAPTER TWO
When is the best time to have a baby?

Just when you thought you had your life under complete control, your sister will announce that she is pregnant, or you will visit your best friend in the maternity ward. Then, out of the blue, it hits you — the baby bug. After years of denying to yourself and to everyone else, for that matter, that you were the slightest bit interested in children, cracks will appear in your highly enamelled and polished external image and a 'soft' centre will start to exert a gentle and persuasive influence on your career-orientated single mindedness.

You suddenly find yourself drawn to the maternity-wear and baby clothes departments. You start to take more notice of magazine articles about pregnancy. You even buy a book about the subject! This behaviour is a sure sign that after having long been subjugated to ambition, your maternal instincts are at last starting to assert themselves.

But, somewhere inside, the 'corporate you' will speak up, loud and long. 'I can't possibly have a baby next year. We're right in the middle of our new product launch.' 'I'm going to have to travel to Europe at least once a month.' 'I wouldn't dare hand this project over to anyone else,' and, 'After all I've done I don't want to.' Anyway, how on earth would I break the news to my clients and the office.' 'I'm just about to be offered a seat on the board. I could not possibly jeopardise my career like that.' After discussing it with your partner, you soften up slightly. 'Okay,' you say, 'But it's going to have to wait until I've landed this contract.' (or whatever).

Unfortunately, the sad fact of the matter is that approaching the decision about having a baby on the basis of rational argument gets you nowhere. You will come up with so many good, strong, practical reasons against the idea, that, ultimately, you will find that there is never an ideal time to have a baby. In fact, many women reaching their mid-thirties who have been afraid to take the plunge or unable to decide have been grateful that an 'accidental' pregnancy saved them from actually having to make this momentous decision.

Many others in their twenties and thirties are so caught up in the day-to-day challenges and excitement of their working life that they do not even consider the possibility of children. It is unlikely that they ever come into contact with mothers and babies, since their circle of friends and colleagues is also likely to be childless. But, while they may be very much against the idea of having children in their twenties and early thirties, when they reach late thirties and early forties, they may begin to feel that they have missed out as they see the prospect of ever having a child (let alone children) disappear over the watershed of their fortieth birthday. Suddenly, financial and material success seem trivial and empty, and the goals they set out to achieve in their twenties without fundamental value and basically unrewarding in comparison to having a child. It is as if the struggle to achieve recognition and career success were more fulfilling than actually being at the top. Perhaps it is just the effect of the wisdom of age and experience, but what seems like a glamorous, satisfying way of life when you are 25 may prove to be surprisingly unfulfilling when you are 45, because of boredom and repetition, because actually being a director is less exciting than you imagined, or simply because you become more realistic about what matters in life. Acquiring more money and material possessions for their own sake seems less important when you already have a high standard of living and quality of life. Constantly battling to retain your position and maintain your performance to the highly tuned model of efficiency you have created for yourself may become very tiring and really not worth the effort.

Even though you may be confident about your negative views on children *now*, it is important to be at least aware of the way the desire to be a mother may creep up on you unexpectedly, releasing emotions and psychological pressures which will surprise you by their power.

Coupled with this emotional pressure is a sudden rise in fertility at about the age of 39. So any ambivalence towards having babies and chances taken with contraception could result in an unexpected pregnancy.

And that isn't all — babies are in fashion nowadays. *Everyone* is having them. Films and television programmes are being made about motherhood and fatherhood and about the new breed of working mother. Career girls are being made to feel that instead of a company Porsche, what they *really* need as a symbol of their success is a baby, proof positive that they have achieved the twin goals of motherhood and a career. It is not enough any more to be just a high-achiever at work. That's easy

— you can devote yourself to your job in the same way a man can. *Real success* is combining the roles of career woman and mother successfully, or so it would appear if you examine the implications of the sudden upsurge of interest in babies.

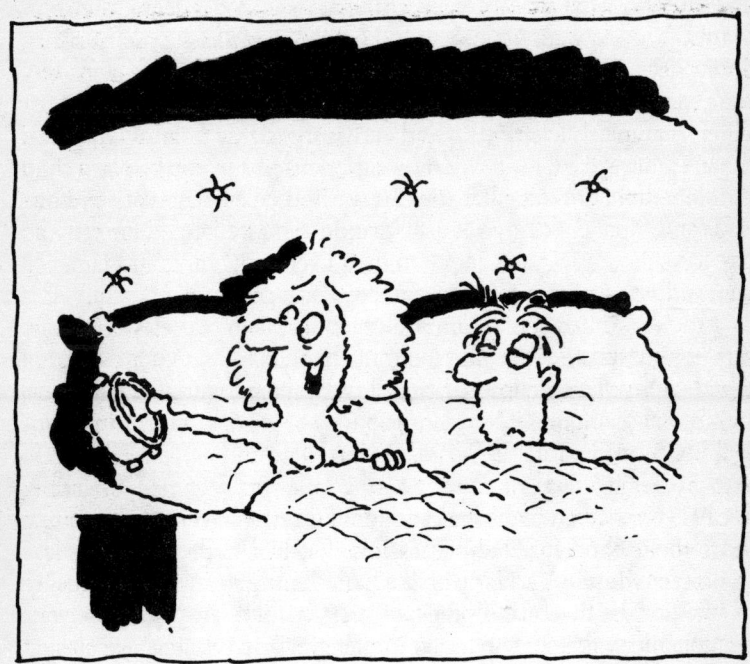

So, when is the best time to have a first baby and join the ranks of parenthood, one of life's most unpredictable and demanding of roles?

The first thing is to think about what you mean by 'best'! Is that best for your own emotional and physical well-being? Best for your job or career? Best for your relationship with your husband/partner? Best economically and domestically? Or best for the health and welfare of your baby?

If your motive for continuing to work after your marriage is purely financial, and you are primarily interested in a salary rather than a career, you will probably be of the opinion that the timing of motherhood will be a question of 'simple' economics. However, you may find that it isn't as simple as all that! Financial hurdles keep cropping up. Paying off the loan for the car, having one last summer holiday together, moving to a bigger house, waiting until your partner gets that promotion can all seem like perfectly good excuses for putting off having a baby for another six months. The fact is that there isn't going to be any ideal time to have a baby from a purely financial point of view. This can be especially true as, when the time comes, you might find that you are more reluctant than you think to give up your financial independence and freedom to do what you want when you want to. Having to ask your husband for money and justify your domestic expenditure might be more painful and demoralizing than you imagined, as can having to formulate a major plan of campaign to move more than a hundred yards from your front door. There will be no more nipping round to the corner shop for a pint of milk or deciding that you can't be bothered to cook one evening and eating out. The degree of organization and foresight required in the day-to-day 'running' of a baby can be quite intimidating, and is just as demanding as running a department of a large company.

However, women with an ambivalent attitude to motherhood, or more serious ambitions, may want to evaluate the pros and cons of having a baby when they are in their twenties compared with when they are a primeval sounding 'elderly primagravida' — as the maternity clinics will insist on describing you at 30 plus.

There is no doubt that the best biological time for a woman to have her first baby is between 20 and 30, when, statistically, there appear to be fewer complications and the greatest chance of having a normal baby. However, if the potential mother is newly married, the chances are her relationship with her husband will not be very well established. Having a baby at this time can put a huge strain on any couple, let alone on a relatively immature marriage. Couples who become parents before they have had time to spend together as husband and wife may find themselves unsettled by the dramatic changes in their lifestyle coming so soon one after the other, without time to absorb the implications of these changes. Similarly, couples who decide to have a baby to cement a rocky relationship should be aware that they are only adding to the stress factors already dogging their relationship and could be speeding up the breakdown of their marriage.

A young mother may well have more stamina and energy to carry her through pregnancy and the stressful early weeks after the baby is born. But what she gains in terms of physical strength, she may lack in emotional maturity and find herself succumbing more easily than an older women to the negative aspects of motherhood such as loss of freedom, increased responsibility, and the constant demands made on her by her baby. She sees her husband free to enjoy the independence and social aspects of his job. Perhaps he travels away from home, or works long hours while she is left at home all day to cope with the baby. This can lead her to resent the baby and increase her sense of isolation from the real world. In marriages where the wife has stayed at home from the beginning to be a traditional wife and bring up the children, the couple may even grow apart as the husband ascends the corporate hierarchy while she remains 'just a housewife'.

Women in their early twenties will not yet have had time to establish a track record in their job or career, or, even to have made up their mind exactly what they want to do with their life, which may make it more difficult for them to return to work if they decide to stay at home for more than two or three months. This is because they may not have been in their jobs long enough to qualify for statutory maternity leave, nor to expect their employer to make special provision to allow them to return to work.

Unless she returns to some form of education or retraining once the children are at school and makes a completely fresh start, a woman who has started her family young seems to lose out in the job market and has to fight harder for acceptance than the better established older woman. She may well be rejected automatically in any future job application if she has not worked for a number of years because her skills are no longer current. Even in the traditional career of secretary, for example, the rapid development of office technology means that she will have been left far behind in the skills race, and will need retraining. The qualities of determination and ability will be just as important for the woman returning to work after having children as a woman who puts her career first. She will have to fight just as hard for recognition, and may have to fight even harder against deep-rooted prejudice which automatically rules that married women returning to work are second best!

However, some employers are finding that women returning to work at more mature ages, having brought up their families, have more to offer by way of self-motivation, organizational skills and reliability than a younger, less confident and self-assured girl. Nevertheless, the rise in the numbers of women having their first baby at 30-plus, and even in their early forties, would seem to demonstrate a growing recognition of the damage women do to their careers by having their family when they are comparatively young.

This has been helped by developments in gynaecology and the high level of expertise and technology now used in modern obstetrics. Older women can now have their first child at what was once considered to be a dangerous age.

What are the effects of maternal age on the baby? It is true that older mothers are prone to more problems — the most worrying of which is the likelihood of having a Down's syndrome baby, a risk curve which increases with maternal age. The chances of *any* woman having such a child are 1 in 660, according to research figures, but at 20, it is 1 in 2,000, between 30 and 34, 1 in 750, between 35 and 40, 1 in 300, and between 40 and 45, 1 in 45. For over 45s the risk is 1 in 17. Pre-natal screening, usually by amniocentesis, is therefore offered to women automatically after the age of 37, with the option of having an abortion if this or any other defects such as spina bifida are detected. High blood pressure and diabetes may also occur more frequently in women in their mid-30s and older, and the incidence of longer than average labours, induction and the use of forceps may also be increased.

Apart from statistics about the increased risk of having a Down's syndrome baby if you put off childbearing until the 30-40 age bracket, and the possible increase of your chance of conceiving twins, the age of the mother seems to have very little impact on the personality and intelligence of the child.

It is sometimes argued that the 20-year-old mother will be closer and more in tune with her children as they enter into their teens, while an older mother will suffer from a wider generation gap. She may even be claiming her pension before her children have finished their education! Other experts say that a intelligent 40-year-old, professional mother will have a better chance of having an intelligent child than a 20-year-old. Perhaps it is simply a case of the older, career woman, being able to pass on to her child the benefit of her experience and broad knowledge of life.

Older mothers are sometimes said to be more anxious about their baby and more prone to depression. They may feel inadequate at coping with a new baby and isolated at home all day, whereas only a few weeks ago, they were able to manage and motivate a staff of 20 and achieve huge sales and profits, yet their tiny scrap of a child reduces them to a physical and emotional wreck!

Potentially the most worrying problem facing female high-fliers who postpone their first pregnancy until their thirties and beyond is infertility.

Fertility *does* decline with age and can be affected by stress, although the positive stress experienced by working women may not necessarily be harmful. A healthy woman in her early twenties has a 30 per cent chance of becoming pregnant within one month, and an 80 per cent chance of becoming pregnant in a year. A woman between 20 and 25 has a 95 per cent chance of becoming pregnant compared with 89 per cent in the 26-30 bracket, 83 per cent between 31-35 and 76 per cent between 36 to 40. The decline in fertility is comparatively slow until the age of 30, when it accelerates quite rapidly from the age of 35 onwards (with a hiccup around 39 or 40).

If a woman of 38 seems unable to conceive, the most likely response of her GP will be to tell her to wait two years. The NHS will only investigate cases of failure to conceive after this time. Because of a lack of resources, some NHS clinics have a cut off date of 38 or may have long waiting lists. You will also have to go through unofficial vetting procedure, similar to that given to prospective adoptive parents. These time constraints may leave you with the only option of going to the private sector and incurring potentially huge costs, which could be in the range of £100-£10,000, and involve months of tests and treatment. Even here, there is pressure, since success cannot be guaranteed, and you may need to have more than one attempt at the new techniques of artificial insemination, test-tube or new GIFT method before becoming pregnant. Doctors will counsel couples embarking on this kind of treatment about the strain it will place on themselves and their relationship. You should also bear in mind that an obsession with becoming pregnant could also impair your concentration and performance at work.

Women who postpone pregnancy until their late thirties often take failure to conceive particularly badly. Quite apart from the disappointment at not being able to have a child, the high-achiever will often be unfamiliar with failure in *any* sense, and may feel more guilty and resentful than a younger woman would in similar circumstances. She may blame herself unfairly for having literally left it too late.

Yet, in spite of the potential emotional and physical risks of waiting before having children, more and more successful career women are doing just this.

If a woman's infertility cannot be overcome, she may consider adoption. Here again, her age and the fact that she works full-time could be an obstacle.

The availability of babies for adoption is dwindling and couples have to meet strict criteria. Firstly, you have to prove that either you or your partner is infertile. If you are an unmarried couple over 35, or have been married for less than three years, or more than fifteen, the chances are that you will not even be considered as possible adoptive parents.

Quite apart from the stringent routine vetting procedure, a woman who had put her career before children would have her motives for adoption subjected to vigorous examination. Most adoption agencies would be very suspicious of placing a child with such a person, particularly if they felt that the baby would be cared for by a nanny most of the time.

The adoption procedure can also be long and trying, taking as long as nine months, a deliberately contrived timescale to ensure the parents' strong commitment. For a working (potential) mother with a demanding job, the waiting and uncertainty may be too high a price to pay in terms of the increased pressure and conflict of interest she may have to resolve.

Many older women seem to thrive when they are pregnant, particularly if they are carrying a much-wanted baby. Provided she remains fit and healthy during her pregnancy and the baby is developing well, there is no physical reason why a woman of whatever age should not continue to work until quite late into her pregnancy, as long as she tries to fit in as much rest as possible and respects her condition. This is particularly easy with a first baby, since there are fewer demands on her out of work hours.

French doctors have found that women in 'boring' jobs are twice as likely to have premature babies as those with 'stressful' but stimulating and varied occupations. British doctors intend to look into the effects of working on a pregnant woman, and will take into account such factors as travelling to work, as well as the environmental conditions in the case of factory workers or laboratory staff. Fear of unemployment as a result of pregnancy should not be overlooked as a potential source of stress for women who are dependent on their salary.

Doctors agree that it would be helpful if they could determine whether, by giving up work at, say 28 weeks, women could seriously improve their chances of a normal birth, or alternatively, that there was no apparent harm in working until they could no longer fit comfortably in the office lift or behind their desk.

Post-natal tiredness and the effects of sleep deprivation may be more pronounced in the 30 to 40 year old age group than with younger mothers, but the older mother will generally be less resentful of the time she spends with her children, and may have a more realistic expectation of the fulfilment to be enjoyed from motherhood.

Older parents will also have achieved a higher standard of living and will be emotionally and financially more secure and thus be able to offer a better material standard of living. An older mother will have more to offer her child from her own wider experience of life and from her own confidence and conviction in herself and her achievements. Double-income, older parents will probably be in the fortunate position of being able to afford to indulge their baby, and their own childhood fantasies, in a designer nursery, with hand-painted cribs and furniture and stencilled walls and the most fashionable baby wardrobe, instead of having to be content with the basics from the high-street chainstores.

The pregnant high-flier may also have the money to enable her to have her baby in luxury at one of the private maternity clinics, with the personal attention of a top gynaecologist who can hold her hand and even time the delivery to suit her diary, insofar as this is medically advisable.

In career terms, the 30- or 40-year-old high-achiever will have many more choices open to her. Because she will have proved her worth both to her employer and her clients, she will be in a much stronger position to negotiate the terms of her maternity leave, because her employer will readily recognize the value of her experience and ability.

On the other hand, if you are sure that you want to return to work

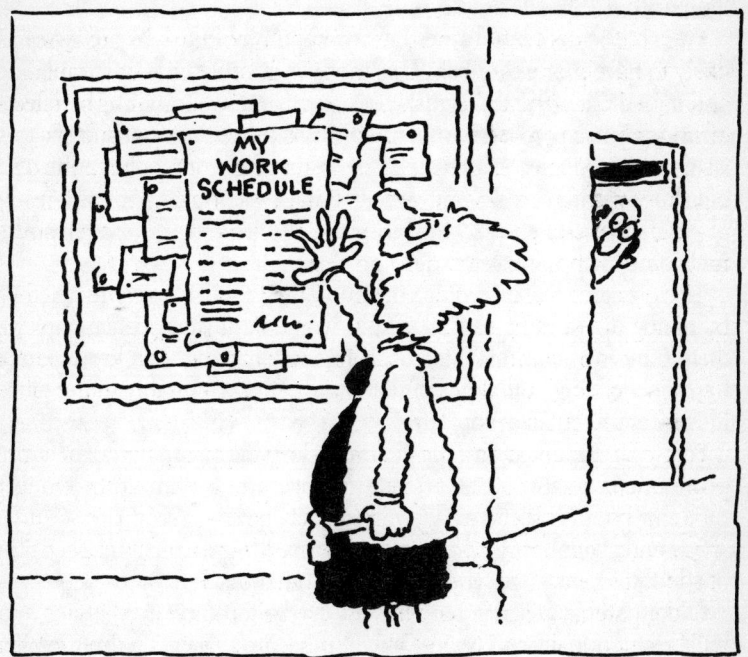

after a short break, you would be wise to plan your pregnancy for a time when you have your job under control, or when it would be convenient to mark time in your career, especially if you plan to take as much maternity leave as possible. You will feel much more relaxed knowing that your temporary absence from the office is causing minimum disruption. It will also help you feel more confident when you tell the office if you have made careful plans about how long you intend to be away, and when.

Such is the intense competitive pressure that exists for many successful women who have made it to the top that they feel compelled to return to their desk as soon as possible after the birth. Never having spent prolonged periods at home, they behave as though they are adrenalin addicts and fear being unable to function out of the highly charged atmosphere of their working environment. However, they may be surprised by their reaction once the baby is born. A new scale of priorities puts a different perspective on work demands. They may even regret having committed themselves to no more than a few weeks' leave.

This can set up a train of unsettling conflict and an acute sense of divided loyalties and the discomfort of being emotionally pulled in different directions at once.

However, the successful career woman is in the fortunate position of having another choice. Because of her experience, confidence and contacts, she is able to think about alternatives to returning to work such as working part-time or trying to develop a business as a freelance consultant, or to set up her own company, perhaps working from home initially. Nevertheless, you should not underestimate the amount of work and attention to detail required to set up a new business, no matter how small, if you are going to get it off the ground successfully. Trying to embark on a new enterprise, or even to organize freelance assignments in late pregnancy or shortly after the baby is born could prove difficult, as it is incredible how little time there is in the first few months to do anything other than change nappies, do the laundry, eat and sleep.

Ideally you should have at least done the groundwork of a new business or freelance career, say a year before becoming pregnant, and have developed it to a stage where you can withdraw your full-time involvement and allow yourself some time to concentrate on the baby. It would be foolish to leave full-time work to give yourself more freedom to enjoy your baby, only to find you are even more pressured by the equally demanding fledgling business you are trying to nurture.

Some senior female executives may finally admit that what they would like is a complete break from the pressures of work and actually decide, either to take a sabbatical and return to work as much as 18 months later, if this can be arranged, or to opt out of business completely to bring up the child themselves. Having fulfilled their career objectives, there are no longer any challenges to be met, and motherhood and domesticity may appear to provide a welcome alternative. It is ironic that this is exactly the reverse of the situation faced by generations of women for whom work provided an escape from the inevitable claustrophobia of family life.

It is important to try to keep your options open about your return to work. Just because the media supermums leave their desks the day before they have the baby and return a week later, you should not be forced into a similar course of action to prove how indispensable you are. You will be putting yourself under a lot of strain from which, ultimately, it will take you longer to recover and which will make you ill at ease with yourself, and difficult to live and work with.

If you do decide to return to work within such a short timescale, you will have little option but to hand over the new baby almost completely to the care of a nanny, both day and night, and, most probably, forego the important bonding process of feeding the baby yourself. However, if you can spend at least three or four months getting to know your baby, you should be able to establish a strong mother-child relationship and prevent future identity/role conflicts between yourself and whoever is looking after the baby.

It is important to think about what kind of a mother you want to be and what you expect from your relationship with your child *before* you decide on the best course of action. If you get off on the wrong foot working when you rather wouldn't, or vice versa, it could take you a long time to get on the right track, and you could risk a great deal of emotional hardship while you are getting there.

How does the 'best time' criterion apply to your relationship with your husband or partner? In most cases, the father will find that he has been relegated to the bottom division in your scale of priorities in the first few months after you have your baby.

If you are in your twenties and newly married, your husband may find it difficult to accept the demands made on your time and feel jealous of your relationship with the baby. If you have been together for a number of years, though, you will have established a strong rapport and understanding to be able to cope. And if you have already worked fairly long hours in a demanding job, the chances are that your husband will be used to helping out around the house and would be as surprised to come home to find you preparing a romantic candle-lit supper after you've had the baby as he would have been before. Even before children, most successful double-income marriages are based on a domestic partnership, otherwise they would have foundered long ago. With the experience of taking on his share of the housework, the older father may well be more sympathetic and supportive when the new baby arrives. Many couples find that this new dimension in their lives brings them even closer together.

However, if your partner has been used to you being responsible for running the house as well as working, don't expect him to change overnight. Unlike women who are adept at juggling priorities and adapting to new situations, the first-time, older father may have become too set in his ways to be as helpful as you would like.

How many children you want is also an important factor in deciding when to have the first baby. Many women have two children close together, taking a career break of as much as seven years, and then returning to work as soon as possible. Other working women prefer to space the children out, with three–five year gaps between each one, returning to work after three–four months' maternity leave after each baby, progressing their career a stage further before taking another period of maternity leave a few years later.

There are no easy answers to the timing of having a baby. Only you can make such a personal decision. It will all come down in the end to how much you want to have a baby, or whether you feel in your heart of hearts that being a mother is not for you just yet. If you *do* decide to have a child, the route you will take as a working mother will take you over a series of emotional and physical hurdles of Olympic proportions, but you will be astounded by your ability to negotiate them successfully, and by the fulfilment doing this will give you.

CHAPTER THREE
Coping with motherhood

'No one told me it would be such hard work.' 'If only I could get some sleep, I would be able to cope.' I used to think my job was demanding.' 'The day just passes me by in a haze of feeding and changing.' 'I look and feel terrible and the house is a complete mess.'

These comments are typical of many first-time mothers, particularly if they long entertained notions of perfect motherhood and have delayed having children until their thirties or early forties.

No training course could ever be designed to prepare a woman for the challenge of being a mother. And even though, deep down, you are overjoyed at having produced a much-wanted and healthy baby, you might be in for a shock at the sheer hard work of keeping a baby clean and fed in the first few weeks. It is important to realize that you are not the only new mother to feel this way. It happens to everyone.

If you had a trouble-free pregnancy and worked up to the last minute, without giving yourself time to slow down or adjust to the idea of impending motherhood, you will probably be even less prepared for the effects of being literally thrown into such a chaotic and demanding role without any transition from the relatively ordered world of work. Even if you left work six weeks or a month before, you will still be reeling from the shock of the relentless demands made on you by the baby. On the whole, first-time mothers are so anxious about how they will cope with labour and the delivery that they spend months reading books and attending classes to prepare themselves mentally and physically for this experience, forgetting that this is only the beginning. They become so preoccupied with the excitement of becoming pregnant and the experience of labour, it comes as quite a shock to realize that this is not the end, and that, in fact, the real job of motherhood only begins once the baby is born.

How you react to being a first-time mother will depend on a number of factors: how long you have worked and how successful you have been in achieving your ambitions; how long you have waited for a baby; whether or not you had difficulty in conceiving; what kind of pregnancy or labour you expected and experienced; the sex of the baby. All these factors will combine with post-natal exhaustion and the natural anxiety about the new baby to leave you wondering what on earth ever inspired you to have this baby anyway. And where is the overwhelming maternal love you were expecting to feel? If only you could get some sleep. Never before has any job made such demands on your stamina.

Younger mothers are probably better equipped to cope with the disruption of having a very small baby, being more flexible and having more stamina. Older mothers tend to be more set in their ways and used to controlling every aspect of their lives. You had probably never believed friends who warned you about the after-effects of having a baby. You were sure that they were exaggerating and that with your proven organizational skills and training, you would sail through the early days.

Media reports about the dynamic super-career-mother who leaves her office the day before to have a pre-arranged, induced birth to return a week later to take up exactly where she left off do a great disservice to most working women who feel a sense of abysmal failure and wonder why they are still in their dressing gown at lunch-time, trying to find the time to do last night's washing up. For years, immaculately groomed and in complete control of their lives, they have put in a twelve-hour day; now the simplest of domestic chores takes up all their time. One new mother summed up the situation well when she explained that for her, to have bathed and dressed herself and the baby by the end of the day was a major achievement. For women used to taking in their stride whatever the working day threw at them, this can be extremely frustrating and depressing. Whereas once you used to be able to juggle three phone calls at once, trying to make a personal phone call is now a major undertaking requiring skill and determination.

One of the commonest emotional problems to which new mothers are prone is post-natal depression. It is no respecter of persons and can strike successful professional women in their luxury nurseries surrounded by loving husbands and all the domestic support they need as easily as a single, unmarried mother living in a high-rise block on social security. Like the desire to become a mother, its origins are unknown but are thought to lie deep in the recesses of the female emotional and hormonal make-up.

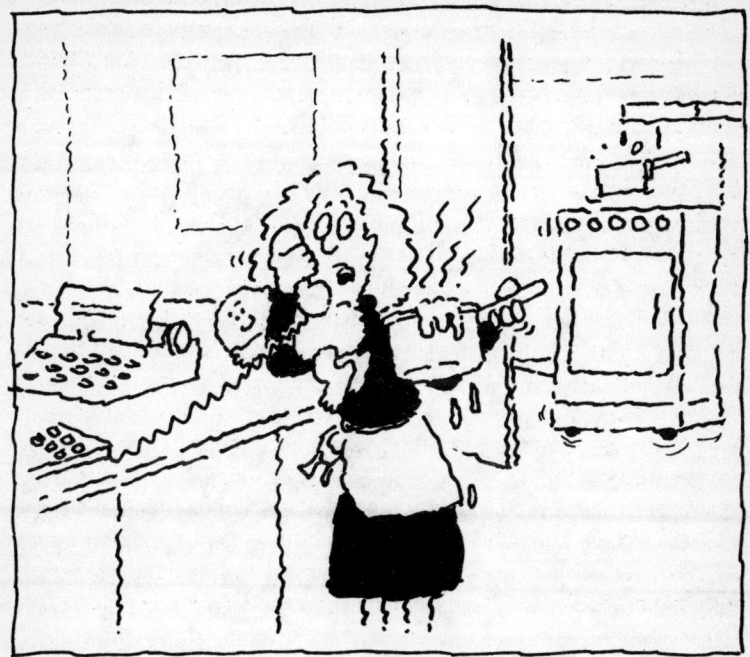

Between 10 and 15 per cent of women experience a depressive illness after childbirth, and at least half have not recovered by the time the child has reached its first birthday. Full-strength post-natal depression is not to be confused with the 'baby blues' and tearfulness that may present itself around the third day after the delivery when the milk comes in and it disappears soon afterwards. Fortunately only about 1 in 1,000 mothers suffer from chronic depression lasting more than a year.

The high-flying executive who goes through her pregnancy convinced that she can schedule motherhood into her life like another business appointment may be most prone to depression when she realizes how impossible this will be. It is the loss of structure and routine in the lives of these women that hits them hardest and subjects them to considerable strain.

Depression and anxiety may also arise out of sheer loneliness and isolation. An older mother may not have many friends who have children the same age as hers and, if they have worked throughout the pregnancy, will not have met many other new mothers before the baby was born. Many women in this position find it difficult to meet other mothers with whom they have anything in common at mother and baby clinics for example, especially if they return to work soon after the birth. The working mother may be made to feel inadequate and heartless by the remarks of women who are taking a prolonged break from work, and may often find their resolve challenged by their own emotional response to such criticism.

Apart from clinical post-natal depression and anxiety, one of the most probable reasons why the perfectionist executive woman may suffer from feeling generally down after the birth is a strong sense of anti-climax. Everyone else — doctors, nurses, health visitors, family and friends — troop through the house to admire baby, and expect mother to feel ecstatic and elated. She knows she ought to be feeling this way, but instead she feels depressed, disappointed, exhausted and anxious. Where is the sudden rush of maternal love? After all, she has waited long enough to have this baby and yet, somehow, it is not at all how she imagined it would be. Instead of joy and exhilaration, she feels as though her brain has been turned into so much scrambled egg as she floats, shell-shocked from the whole experience of late pregnancy and labour through the whole gamut of post-natal emotions. It is all she can do to concentrate long enough to fill in the daily hospital menu card in time for it to be collected. One such mother, afraid that her brain had completely disintegrated never to reactivate again, asked her husband to bring the *Financial Times* into hospital each day, only to have it lie, unopened, at the end of the bed, a sharp reminder of her former mental powers.

You were probably aware of a degree of amnesia and vagueness during the later half of your pregnancy, as your energies seemed to drain from your intellect to support the growing baby. It is all part of nature's efforts to render you calm, impassive and serene so that you drift through the whole experience without too much resistance to the displacement of your reason by your emotions. Unfortunately, this can be very disconcerting for the manager or executive used to making split-second decisions and she will be somewhat alarmed at the loss of her mental agility. Instead of taking everything as it comes, she will fight against this temporary loss of brain power, fearing it may be permanent. After all, she depends upon her intellectual ability to earn her living as much as the athlete or opera singer depends on physical strength or voice. So it is in the early weeks after the baby arrives that the first-time executive mother feels at her most vulnerable. How could she ever have been so foolish as to imagine that she could ever return to work, let alone allow anyone else to look after the baby?

It is very important that you don't try to analyse your feelings too much nor make any irrevocable decisions at this point. It is much wiser to postpone any changes in your original plan until you have emerged from the cocoon of pregnancy, as you undoubtedly will, a bit bruised and battered, but a great deal stronger as a result of the transformation into a mother. Many first-time mothers are surprised by the beneficial effects on their personality. Those who tended to be somewhat diffident before, often find it easier to become more assertive and have an increased sense of confidence and fulfilment and those who were rather aggressive or abrasive become a lot more mellow and 'laid back'. Perhaps it is just that being responsible for a child acts as a yardstick against which other priorities, job pressures and challenges are measured and evaluated. What would have caused a major crisis before the baby, may seem rather trivial and unimportant once the threshold into parenthood has been crossed. Some women, who have been absolutely certain of their intention to return to work after having a child, find their feelings towards the baby so overwhelming that they abandon the idea of going back to their job and give it all up to stay at home.

Women who persevere and do return to work find that coming home at night to a baby and the relaxation of the bath and bedtime routine helps them switch off from the day's pressures and they are able to leave their worries about work behind them at the office. So grateful are most new mothers for a night's sleep that the most serious problem in the office will never be allowed to disturb their much-needed rest.

Many new mothers are also surprised by the way they find hidden depths to cope with the dual pressures of a baby and a job. Sleep deprivation is the worst problem and difficult to cope with if you have a baby who is unable to sleep through the night until it's quite old. One mother who frequently travelled to Europe on business sometimes found that she was getting into bed at 3.30 am, having spent almost an hour awake coping with the baby, only to have to get up at 5 am to catch an early morning flight. Somehow, she would get through the day, in a dream-like state, only to collapse on the return flight home and snatch an hour's sleep.

Most babies and young children develop an irritating knack of disturbing you the night before an important meeting, but working mothers learn to cope with this inevitable problem very quickly. Of course, if they have a live-in nanny, they can organize it so that they do not have to wake up. But many mothers feel that they ought to cope with the child at night to ensure the continuing strength of their parent-child bond and make up in some way for their absence during the day.

Most working mothers will push themselves to the limits of their endurance in their attempts to spend as much time with their children when they are not working in order to fend off the most persistent and recurring of problems to which all working mothers are prone — guilt.

It is all-pervasive. When you are working, you feel guilty that you are not spending time with your children, when you take time off work to be with your children, you feel guilty about not being in the office.

One experienced working mother has learned to come to terms with this most powerful of emotions: 'Once a working mother accepts that guilt is an inevitable and inescapable part of her existence, she will be half way to coping with it and learning to live with it.' A working mother should never forget that even when previous generations of women stayed at home to look after the family, their time was not usually devoted to reading and playing with the children. There was a house to run, washing to be done, clothes to be ironed, food to be bought and prepared. In the days before domestic gadgetry and time-saving appliances, this took up most of the day and, even now, this still takes up the larger part of the non-working mother's time. Working mothers are wrong when they assume that women who stay at home spend all day with the children. The children are simply fitted in around the day's chores.

Even when she realizes this, to make up for the time she is away from her children, the working mother will very often overcompensate by giving what the child experts now term 'quality time' to their children. Most children of working mothers very soon learn to understand that mummy works, and, ironically, are often very proud of them.

The most testing time is undoubtedly in the early months of your return to work, when the baby is still very young and you are not completely confident about the strength of the baby's own relationship with you. 'Will he prefer the nanny?' is the most common question asked by working mothers at this time, and, indeed, many diehard career girls flinch visibly when they come through the front door to find a picture of maternal perfection starring their nanny and child. At times like this, maternal jealousy and anxiety can rock you to the very core and you will doubt the wisdom of what you are doing with your life. However, if you have established a strong bond with your child in the first few weeks, you will be reassured that, in spite of your daily absence, it is *you* he will seek out when he is tired or ill. For there is no way you can deny the fundamental relationship between mother and child. And unless you have handed over to someone else the emotional as well as the physical care of your child, you need not fear for their love.

In fact, in most cases, it is not the child, but the mother who suffers most. Older mothers have an added disadvantage in that they are possibly too idealistic about the pleasures of motherhood. The working mother tends to overanalyse many of the situations she finds herself in, running to consult books, only to find that in most cases, answers cannot be found. The executive woman is so used to gaining her knowledge and experience from the textbook, the manual, the professional procedure, that she feels an alien in the world of motherhood, where so much is governed by instinct. The modern executive woman, however, has probably worked hard at subjugating her maternal instinct to the pursuit of ambition and the extension of her intellectual capacity. She has to dig deep to re-discover her instincts and then has to have the confidence to trust them where her own child is concerned. This is why the mother who is a high achiever in her career will usually enjoy her second child more than the first, having adjusted to the demands and developed the skills being a mother requires.

It is also important to follow your own instincts about your own child and not be lead by the many conflicting views you will hear about how to bring up a baby. If you and your child have fallen into a routine you're both happy with, don't, under any circumstances, be persuaded to change it.

As the first, and most traumatic, phase of motherhood draws to a conclusion towards the end of the second month, you will begin to see the light at the end of the tunnel and begin to feel strong enough to face going back to work. Don't feel guilty about looking forward to this return. Quite apart from economic necessity, many women need the mental and social stimulus of their job to keep them going. It would be dangerous to deny yourself the choice and end up feeling resentful and trapped by the child and domesticity. A mother who is self-confident, fulfilled and happy will be a better mother than someone who resents her baby for taking away her independence.

Despite your initial anxieties and emotions, by the time you have spent three or four months looking after the baby yourself, and are beginning to enjoy the baby and its growing responsiveness to you, you will be surprised about how strange you now feel leaving the baby behind to go to work each day. No matter how much you enjoy your job, you will find your mind wandering back to the baby and its routines. One new mother used to add up how many hours a week she spent with the baby compared with the nanny, and was only really happy in the office when she knew the baby would be asleep anyway.

If you can phase your return to work gradually, it will give you time to adjust to leaving the baby in the care of someone else. If you can arrange to work, say, part-time or on flexi-time, it will also help you adjust to the new pace of life. It is not a bad idea to arrive home unexpectedly once or twice so that you can judge first-hand the way in which the baby is being looked after when you are not there.

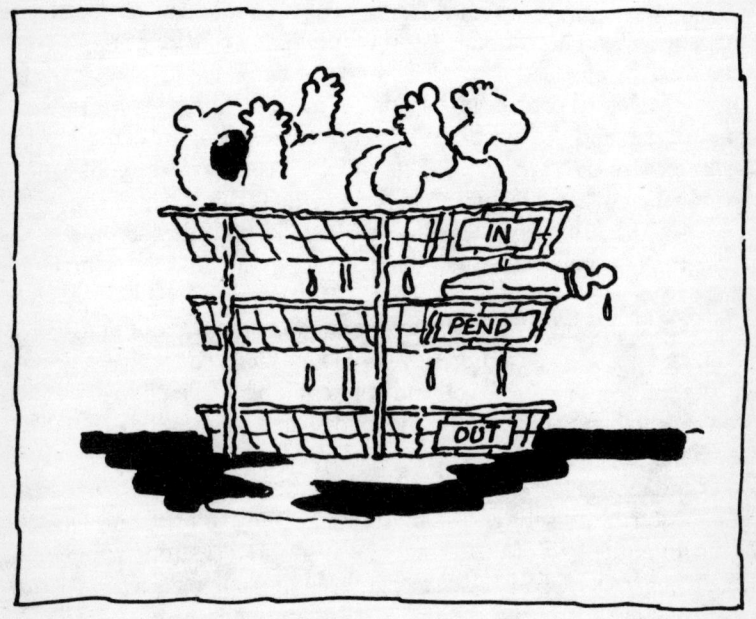

Having a baby will mean the greatest upheaval in your life. Being used to handling the challenges of their working life makes it all the harder for older, working mothers to accept these changes. Everyone will react differently to being a mother for the first time. It may be that you will feel the exact opposite of what you expected. The older mother who is having an unplanned pregnancy may be overwhelmed by the experience and fall in love with her baby immediately. Another mother, who has orchestrated her pregnancy and her return to work with precision, may be disappointed and disillusioned that being a mother was not as she had foreseen it.

No matter how difficult those early months are, the best advice offered by a full-time career mother who ran a successful publishing company was that, no matter how difficult it is at the time, you should not lose sight of the fact that much of it can be regarded as just another phase in the development of the child, *and* in your response to it. None of them lasts for ever, and by the time the baby is three, you will be delighted by the companionship, humour, love and fun you experience with your child.

CHAPTER FOUR
Child-care and the working mother

Once you know you are pregnant and you have made your mind up to return to work after a period of maternity leave, the most important decision you will have to make is who will look after the baby while you are at the office.

The lack of reliable child-care is frequently cited as one of the main reasons women do not return to their old job, or opt for part-time work. Indeed, the UK lags far behind other European countries in allowances for parental leave — that is, leave for both parents — or, indeed, in the provision of any other forms of child-care for working parents.

It is very easy to underestimate the importance of choosing the right person, or the best child-care arrangement. Many pregnant, would-be working mothers say, confidently 'Well, of course, I will just get a nanny and come back to work after three or four months'. 'Just getting a nanny', or anyone else for that matter, to care for your child might prove a lot more difficult than you think, not least because of how you will feel about your baby once it arrives. It is hard to imagine beforehand just how strong your protective, maternal instincts will be, and how great a part your emotions will play in your choice of someone to look after your baby.

It is vital for a mother returning to work to be completely happy about the arrangements she makes for her child. If she is not, her performance at work will suffer and her relationship with her child will become strained. If you are unlucky enough to make a mistake, it will not only be disruptive and unsettling for the baby, it will damage your own confidence and call into question the feasibility of being a working mother. So, do not be misled, choosing the right person to care for your child will be the single most important factor in your being able both to return to work at all, and to work effectively, and with peace of mind. However, although the newspapers regularly splash the nanny disasters of well-known personalities over their front pages, or carry long exposés of the horror stories of babies and children left in the care of unsuitable and irresponsible trained, and untrained, nannies and childminders, these are very much the exception to the rule. Against these, there are many very contented babies, left in the care of highly competent, and caring women, who form strong attachments to the children and the family, and who provide an excellent, high standard of care. Don't be prejudiced by what you read and are told. As with everything else connected with bringing up children, everyone believes they are an expert. Your best strategy is therefore to be confident and trust your judgement about what is best for your circumstances.

Even when you are satisfied with your nanny or childminder, be prepared for days when your whole support system will collapse, through illness or accident. It is only then, when the nanny has gone down with severe glandular fever or your child is sent home from the nursery with chickenpox, that you will finally realize, in case you have not already done so, that ultimate responsibility for caring for your child falls to you. It may be acceptable for father to return early from Tokyo to attend the carol concert or Open Day. But on days of more mundane domestic crisis, it is the mother who is expected to reorganize her busy schedule and cope with the conflicting demands of work, child, nanny and husband. It is on days such as these that you will find hidden resources of stamina, patience, tact, diplomacy and organizational skills which you would never have believed were in you before you became a mother.

The most difficult period for mothers who work is from the time the baby is born until they reach the age of four, rising five. This is the period when a working mother experiences the most guilt and anxiety that, in spite of her determination to follow her career, she might, after all she has said, be missing out on the child's development: first steps, first words, or other milestones. That is why it is very important to have a good rapport with whoever is looking after your child so that they will be sensitive and aware of these anxieties and ensure that you are kept as close as possible to your child's daily activities and behaviour.

After the age of five, your child will be at full-time school, although he may well have attended a day nursery before then, and your child-care needs will change quite significantly.

So what are the options open to you during the pre-schools years, at least?

Basically, it comes down to what you can afford, or are prepared to pay, whether you think you need full-time or part-time help, and whether

Live-in nanny

At the top of the child-care scale is the trained, live-in nanny, employed for the exclusive care of your child in your own home, within the conditions and expectations agreed from the start. The crème de la crème of the nannying profession are the Norland nannies, trained at the exclusive Norland Nursery Training College, and those who have studied at the Princess Christian college, as they are specifically trained as sole-charge, residential nannies.

However, most nannies will have the NNEB (National Nursery Examination Board) qualification. This is a two-year course run at colleges of further education. There is also the equivalent, but less common, NAMCW (National Association of Maternal and Child Welfare) scheme.

These girls (they usually start the course at 16 or 17) are essentially trained to staff state-run or private day nurseries, but with the decline of this sector of pre-school education, most start their careers as residential nannies, perhaps moving on to work in a nursery, or even start their own, after two or three years' experience of sole charge.

Although Norland and Princess Christian nannies generally wear uniforms, a modern nanny is very different from the traditional image. She is likely to wear jeans and will probably expect to call you by your first name, with your permission, of course. You may wish to keep your distance, but most mothers find that establishing a good rapport with their nanny makes for a better motivated and happier girl and, therefore, a more contented child and a satisfied and trusting mother. A lot of first-time mothers are against the idea of a nanny, still believing that she will take over the child so completely that you will have to ask her permission to enter the nursery. This is far from the reality of today's young professional, who will work *with* you not *against* you in the care of your baby.

The advantages of a live-in nanny who stays with you for at least a year are obvious. Your child will benefit from a one-to-one, stable relationship and you will be able to influence how he spends his time, what he eats, and what sort of stimulus he receives. Of course, the key question troubling every first-time mother who goes out to work is, Will the child become closer to the nanny and grow away from his mother?

The answer is, very definitely, no. Unless you choose to hand over a new baby to the sole emotional as well as physical care of a nanny, your baby will always be drawn to you, its mother, particularly if you established or not you think you can cope with someone else living in your house. The options are:

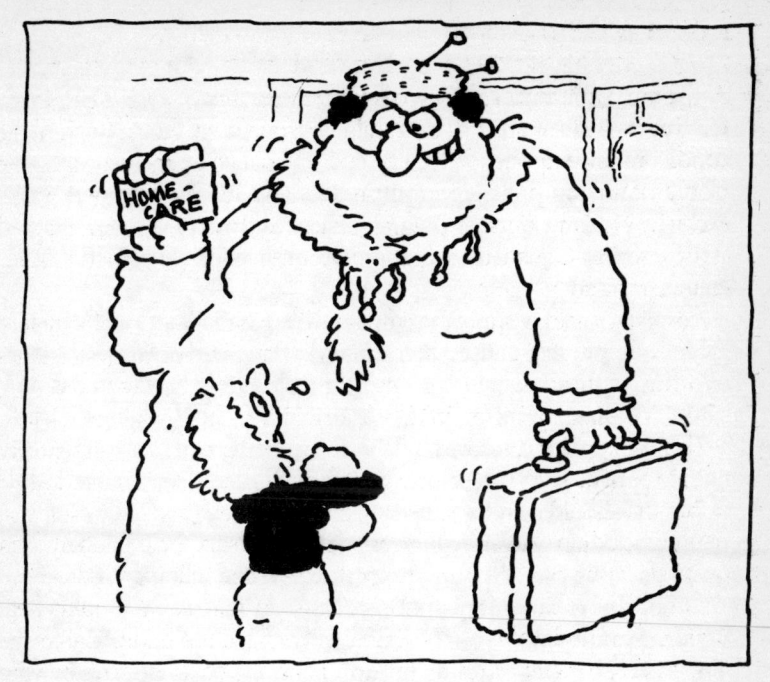

a close bond during your maternity leave, and have breast-fed the child.
　You cannot disturb the fundamental relationship between a mother and child, and nannies are trained to respect the primary importance of your relationship with the child. Those who do try to usurp the role of mother are rare and, if you were to find this tendency developing, you would be well advised to terminate her employment sooner rather than later. It is always a mistake to allow the relationship between you, the nanny and the child to deteriorate to a point where the nanny's departure is fraught with recriminations and bitterness on both sides.
　A nanny will *not* expect to do your ironing, sweep the stairs or wash up your dinner party dishes from the night before. Hers are strictly 'nursery duties only'. The two-year NNEB course covers child development, psychology, nutrition, practical care and creative play and activity. These girls are professional in their approach to their charges and, whatever else you may say about them, having spent two years studying the course and carrying out projects and home placements to gain practical

experience, they have demonstrated a commitment to the task of looking after children. They do not simply become a nanny because they think it is a soft option, better than commuting to an office each day.

Most of the horror stories about nannies are about the relationship with the employer, rather than failure to look after the child properly. Astronomical phone bills, leaving the rubbish bin overflowing every day 'because it is not my job', or leaving the car without petrol after using it for an evening out can all build up tension between you both if not handled properly.

Personality clashes between the employer's expectations and the nanny's performance may also cause a breakdown in their working relationship. Some women find that they are simply unable to tolerate the intrusion of another woman living in their house, no matter how willing the girl may be. Even though you have made it clear from the start that you would prefer the privacy of being alone with your husband in the evenings and that she should be responsible for her own supper and should retire to her own room, you may still feel guilty about her feeling lonely or left out, and this can put a strain on your evening making it hard for you to relax. If your house is not very big, you may not even be able to have a good row with your husband without being overheard. Some couples find that they always end up having a row when the nanny goes out because they know they can 'let go' then. Having a nanny around at the weekends, when she is officially off duty, can also be irritating, especially if she doesn't get up until lunchtime, when you have been up since the crack of dawn with the baby.

Each nanny has her own idiosyncracies. One of mine used so much fabric softener she regularly blocked the washing machine. Another used to turn on the oven as high as it would go for over an hour to bake one tiny egg custard for the baby. At their best, however, nannies are sensitive and caring. One girl turned down her own mother's invitation to bring the baby to join her family for an outing to the zoo because she felt it was the mother's right to take her child to its first day out at the zoo.

If you find the right nanny for you, and there are many excellent nannies around, hang on to her — she will prove to be an absolute gem. Get it right and you will find she will give you a great deal of support, both in and out of the nursery. Most of all, she will give you peace of mind about your child and you will have a contented, secure and well-cared for baby.

If you live in an area where nannies abound, the local 'nanny mafia' can be a wonderful source of back-up if your nanny is away or ill, as they will usually cover for each other in emergency.

There are various ways of finding a nanny. Agencies are a useful source, but they charge a fee which may be refundable if the girl does not work out during a stated minimum period. They tend to attract the more confident, experienced and better qualified nanny, usually looking for a second or third job. You will need to keep nagging them because it is definitely a seller's market, and good nannies are snapped up as soon as they walk through the agency's door. The agency will interview the girl and check her references, but you should satisfy yourself about this by talking to previous employers and checking references yourself. You will find it is not so much what they say, but the way they say it, which is most informative.

You might also try writing to the NNEB Course Tutor at your local college of further education who will advertise your job among her students and will gladly discuss any applicants' qualities with you frankly. A college leaver (they are usually available from mid-June) will be keen and anxious to do her best, but some need some initial direction and guidance. If you find a girl with the right temperament, a college leaver can be an excellent first nanny for a young baby and 'grow up' with the child, gaining in confidence and experience as she gets to know the baby. The advantage of college leavers is that they are not stuck in their ways and you will be able to have things done your way without a clash of personalities.

Many nannies use *The Lady* magazine, or even *Nursery World* as the main source of jobs. Your advertisement should include the number and ages of the children, location, hours, whether you require a driver, or whether non-smoker is preferred, and any other special requirements. Box numbers can be used, but they may reduce the number of applicants and, in any case, it is useful to talk to the girls so that you can gain an impression of each one before selecting the most suitable for interview.

You should allow yourself at least three months to find a nanny, particularly if you have set a firm date for your return to work. When you interview prospective nannies, do not just look at her paper qualifications, no matter how impressive. If she has just left college, ring her tutor to get a first-hand appraisal of her qualities. If she is experienced, ring up her previous employers. Very often the girls' family background and her relationship with her own parents will have a significant effect on how she behaves towards you and your child. It is absolutely vital that you share the same views about child-care, diet, manners, behaviour, otherwise you will be doomed from the start, so make sure you discuss such matters at the interview. You should also discuss duties and hours, etc., and even draw up a 'contract' so that you both know right from the beginning what you expect from each other.

Daily nanny

If a live-in nanny is not for you, either through personal choice or because your house is too small to accommodate one, you might find that a daily nanny would suit you better, although it may cost you more. If your hours and the demands of your job are generally predictable, this arrangement should work well. However, if you are frequently late or need to travel abroad, you may not find this so convenient and find yourself paying over the odds for the extra hours your nanny has to work. There is nothing worse than coming home to an irate nanny at the end of the day when you are late home again or, worse still, passing each other coldly in the hallway. You will also need to make arrangements and pay for babysitting in addition. These costs soon mount up if you have an active social life or go away without the baby at weekends. Daily nannies are easy to come by if you live in London or other major cities, but finding one may be a problem in small towns or in rural areas.

Nanny share

If you work part-time, a nanny-share arrangement might suit you very well. The nanny cares for your child and others either in your home or theirs as agreed, and you share the cost of her salary. It is important to have similar views on child-care and how the children should spend their day. The children benefit from having regular playmates, and some mothers feel such an arrangement helps them to feel that, as one mother put it, 'they are still at the sharp end of motherhood, even though they do work. It would be all too easy to ring up from the office and ask the live-in nanny to do the bath-and-bedtime routine because you are going to be late. At least this way, you make sure you see and relate to your child at an important part of his day.'

Local newsagents' windows sometimes carry nanny-share ads if you live in an area favoured by working couples, and the National Childbirth Trust (NCT) Nannyshare register is very helpful.

Mother's help

If you can afford it, and if you are planning to go out to work, even part-time, employing a trained nanny to look after the baby is the best solution. However, if you are working from home, a mother's help could be the answer. As well as looking after the baby, mothers' helps will help with housework and generally take responsibility for the day-to-day running of the house. If you get a competent, experienced mother's help, she might be able to cope very well with a young baby, but, on balance they are better suited to a household where the mother is around most of the time to direct and guide her. You will not have to pay her as much as a nanny.

You could try a combination of advertising in *The Lady* or using the many agencies specializing in mother's helps, who will try to match you with suitable applicants.

Au pairs

Writing in a series of articles on the various forms of child-care (the *Guardian*, 5 November 1987) Michele Hanson described the use of an au pair as 'woman's inhumanity to woman.' And certainly, of all the horror stories one hears about child-care, those of exploitation of au pairs by their employers and of the sheer negligence, irresponsible behaviour and stupidity on the part of the au pairs themselves, this child-care option is fraught with the most serious pitfalls.

An au pair is not a general dogsbody. They are girls, often students, who have come to the UK to learn English. In return for help with their English and accommodation they do light housework, cooking and look after the children. Au pairs should only work for about 20-30 hours per week, attending college for the rest of the time. You may find yourself becoming a surrogate mother, looking after them, coping with their homesickness, loneliness, or, alternatively, listening anxiously for their return in the early hours of the morning. Language difficulties and communication problems, stories of them packing their bags and leaving in the dead of the night abound. However, many families have been very lucky and have had several excellent au pairs. It is not advisable to give an au pair sole charge of a young baby, but this option works quite well in families with school-age children who need someone to be there to let them in and look after them until you get home.

Child minders

Registered childminders are another popular option for working mothers. You take the child to her home every day where it will be looked after with a number of other children, perhaps including her own. The children will be of different ages with a maximum of only three under-fives and only one baby under a year. Your local social services or the National Childminding Association can provide you with a list of names and addresses. Naturally, you will not have as much control over how your child spends his day as you would if he were being cared for in your home, so you will need to be happy with the childminder's basic approach to diet, exercise, discipline, stimulus, play, and safety while your child is in her care.

Day nurseries

There are a number of council-run and private day nurseries which take young babies, but spaces are not always easy to find. The local council will have details of the ones they run, which are mainly for children from problem families and single mothers.

Placing your child in a privately run day nursery can work very well for many women, but there are some points to be borne in mind. Firstly, although day nurseries may seem to be quite cheap on the face of it, you will have to pay for the days the child does not attend for whatever reason. You might also be asked to supply nappies, bottles and food. Secondly, if your child picks up any diseases — measles, mumps, chicken pox — the nursery will ask you to keep him at home — meaning that you will have to stay home with him. Thirdly, nurseries can be very inflexible about what time your child is collected so they may not be a good choice if you often have to work late.

If you do decide to send your child to a day nursery, watch him carefully. If he seems tearful, tetchy or lethargic, it could be that he is unhappy at the nursery. Don't hesitate to take him away if you feel this is the problem.

On the plus side, a good day nursery can be hard to beat — the child is in a happy, social atmosphere, and the mother has a chance to meet others in the same position.

Workplace crèche

Employers are becoming more sympathetic to the idea of workplace crèches and, at the beginning of 1988, one of the leading American banks opened the doors of a crèche in the City of London to their first eager charges and their even more enthusiastic parents. It is run by a professional nursery organization and places are subsidized by the company, whose employees have priority for the places, although it also serves other companies in the area.

Parents are able to pop in at any time during the day. Indeed, the crèche organizers believe that an open-door policy is essential because the parents have to learn to cope with this new situation and need as much integration as the children themselves.

A valuable spin-off for some mothers has been the development of job-share arrangements which mean that they are also able to rotate the crèche place on the days they are working. And, in fact, the greatest demand on places has been from women working part-time.

Employers' resistance to the idea of a workplace crèche is often based on their view that it would only benefit a few of their female employees who already have young children. They overlook just how comforting it would be for any prospective parent to know in advance that their child could be well looked after in a way that would allow them to continue to work afterwards. In fact, many of the applications for this first City crèche came from the male employees opting to take a place on behalf of their wives who were working elsewhere in the City. This experiment has become a model for a number of others which are planned.

As it finally dawns on more employers that an enlightened approach to maternity leave and child-care would prevent the loss of thousands of pounds in training of top female staff, the workplace crèche may become more commonplace.

Caring for the older child

The most crucial stage for any working mother, whether she works full-time, part-time, or freelance, is the first five years. This is when child-care needs are most concentrated and demanding. You could find it helpful to formulate an overall five-year strategy to carry you through this period. You may well be planning to have a second or third baby, so you should take account of this when deciding on the best form of child-care right from the beginning. For example, while a full-time nanny could be a luxury for a five- or six-year-old who is at school most of the time, if you have another baby at home, the nanny's day will be fully occupied with the new baby, but she will also be on hand to look after the older child on his return, help with homework, bath-time, etc.

A mother's help, or au pair could well be the answer if you work part-time and have children of school age, as you will be around to direct them most of the time.

Although a working mother may find her days freer when the children are at school she may find increased pressure on her availability in the early evening. Picking children up from school in the afternoon, being free to attend school meetings and activities, helping with homework are all important for your child and need a mother's involvement, at least for some of the time. Dropping the child off at school on the way to work will make sure you maintain contact with his day and his teacher. Some full-time working mothers may occasionally take a late lunch and pick up the child from school herself, if the location of school, work and home are conveniently sited.

What does child-care cost?

Although, of course, many women who return to work after having a baby would like to have a full-time, live-in nanny, the sort of child-care you actually have very much depends on what you can afford.

It will come as no surprise to learn that a live-in nanny is at the top of the scale as far as cost is concerned. A fully qualified, experienced nanny will expect to be paid a weekly salary of around £75 per week. On to that you will have to add your national insurance contribution as an employer, and make sure that she pays her NI contribution and tax. You should also take into account the cost of providing her with full board and lodging, and, if she is to do her job well, the use of a car, bringing the cost of a nanny per year to between five and six thousand pounds. This clearly puts a nanny out of reach of most women in their twenties. You would need to be earning well in excess of £25,000 to be able to afford it — bearing in mind that this comes out of your taxed income.

When calculating the cost of a nanny, you will have to take into account

CHILD-CARE AND THE WORKING MOTHER

the fact that she won't do any day-to-day domestic housework, and, if you are working full time, you will need to find someone else to do this, adding to the cost of running the household.

Mother's helps are generally less expensive — they usually earn around £40 per week. This salary is low enough to be tax and national insurance exempt. You will have to consider the fact that a mother's help will generally not work weekends and evenings, except by special arrangement.

Private day-nursery fees start at around £35 per week. On to this you will have to add the cost of a daily cleaner and of babysitting during the evenings. Most nurseries insist that you pay for the place, so you will have to pay even if the child doesn't go if you are going to keep the place open. You will usually have to pay for the food and nappies required for the child, unless you decide to supply your own.

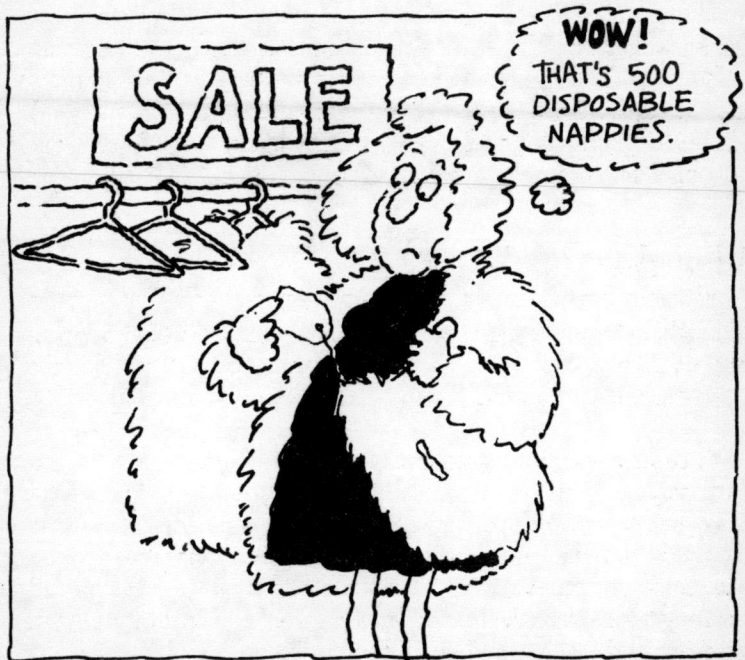

Au pairs' salaries start at around £25 per week, plus board and lodging. It is *not* recommended that you leave a young baby in the sole charge of an au pair.

If you are lucky enough to have a workplace crèche, you will find this is an extremely economic form of child-care. Costs vary from company to company.

Whatever form of child-care you decide to have, your working day will need to be organized with military precision. It has often been said that what every working mother really needs is a wife. Unfortunately, as this is not possible, many working mothers find themselves master-minding a domestic support team of four or five people — she will need to if she is going to have any spare time to spend with her family. As a working mother, you will have to become wife, caterer, nurse, production manager and accountant — all in addition to the demands made upon you by your career — remaining calm, cheerful and controlled at all times. Impossible? You might think so, but most women survive it with their sanity intact, and some even claim to enjoy it!

CHAPTER FIVE
Women and employment

Women now make up over 40 per cent of the workforce, but only 10 per cent approximately are in management and less than 2 per cent are board directors. Over the past decade, recruitment of women into the professions has doubled and, in some cases, trebled. But there is still a long way to go before true equality is realized.

Only 20 per cent of jobs in the professions are held by women, even though as many women as men are now entering solicitors' articles, undergraduate medical training and advertising.

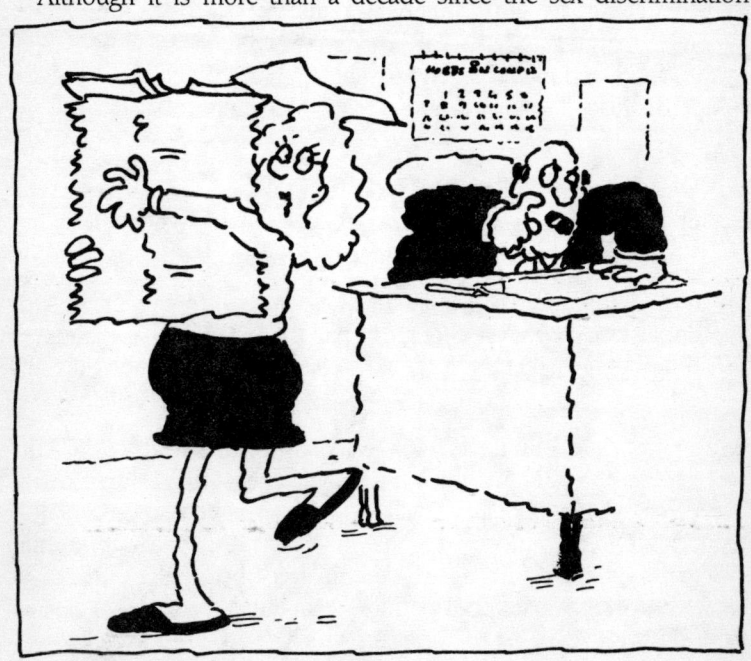

Although it is more than a decade since the sex discrimination legislation came into force in the UK, the practical realization of its prime objective, which was to lift the barriers that prevent women from achieving their full potential alongside men, still has some way to go. There is, however, a growing awareness among employers of the need to formulate an equal opportunities policy, especially among the large public companies.

Yet women still experience what are often described as 'traditional attitudes' towards them on the part of male colleagues. Recruitment and promotion often depend on the attitudes of individual (male) managers, some of whom seem to be more favourably disposed to working women than others.

Whatever the prevailing attitude towards equal opportunities, women still need an employment charter that recognizes and respects, among other things, their right to take maternity leave, or a career break without causing irrevocable long-term damage to their career prospects.

Working women's maternity rights

New rules governing maternity benefits were introduced in 1987 and the new weekly payment, Statutory Maternity Pay (SMP) was introduced by the Government to replace the maternity allowance previously paid by the DHSS, and maternity pay payable from employers. It is paid for up to 18 weeks if you qualify under the following rules:

- You have been employed by the *same* employer for at least 6 months up to the fifteenth week before the week in which the baby is due (i.e. the 26th week of your pregnancy).

- If your employer has dismissed you because you are pregnant and, on average, you earn enough to pay Class 1 National Insurance contributions, you may be treated as satisfying the conditions for SMP.

SMP can be paid for a total of 18 weeks, say from the start of the 11th week before the week in which the baby is due (i.e. the thirtieth week of pregnancy), but it *cannot* be paid for any week in which you continue to work for your employer after that time, so it is up to you to decide whether to stop working at the eleventh week before the birth, or to carry on working up to the last minute. Your entitlement to SMP begins from the week *following* the week in which you cease to work.

As long as you stop work before the start of the sixth week before the week in which the baby is due (i.e. the thirty-fifth week of pregnancy), you can still get payment for the full 18 weeks, but if you work later into your pregnancy, you will lose payment for those extra weeks you work. The amount of SMP you get depends on how long you have worked. If you have been employed continuously for the same employer for at least two years (five years if you work part-time for between eight and 16 hours a week) into the qualifying week, you will receive Statutory Maternity Pay (SMP) payments of 90 per cent of your average weekly earnings for the first six weeks, followed by payments for up to a further 12 weeks at a lower rate. If you have been employed continuously by the same employer for at least six months but less than two years (or less than five years part-time) into the qualifying week, you can receive payments for up to 18 weeks at a lower rate. These rates are reviewed in April each year and can be obtained from the DHSS. You should also note that SMP is treated as earnings, so your employer will make the usual deductions of income tax and NI.

You have to give your employer at least three weeks' notice before you intend to stop work, or as soon as is reasonably practicable. You will also have to give him details of the expected date of birth using Form MAT B1 available from your GP, midwife or maternity clinic.

If you do not qualify for SMP, you may be able to claim maternity allowance from the DHSS if you have a recent work record, and have worked for at least 26 of the last 52 weeks, ending in the fifteenth week before the expected date of confinement. Other benefits such as Income Support or, in some cases, Sickness Benefit, may apply if you do not meet the criteria for the other maternity benefit payments.

SMP must end after 18 weeks, but it may end earlier if you return to work after the baby is born, and before the end of the 18 week period in which SMP is payable. Your contract may entitle you to paid maternity leave at *more* or *less* than SMP, but all employers must at least pay the amounts set out under SMP to all employees who meet the rules.

You should be aware that payment of SMP does not depend on your intending to return to work for your employer after the baby is born, although you may have a right to return to your former job at any time within 29 weeks of your baby's birth if you have worked for the same employer for at least two years. If you do not meet the qualifications, it will be up to your employer to decide whether or not your job will be kept open for your return after maternity leave.

The DHSS publish two booklets setting out the detailed regulations: *Maternity benefits* and *Employment rights for expectant mothers*.

In spring 1988, the CBI issued a statement supporting the principle of equal opportunities in employment. The statement said that the CBI 'favours the application by companies of constructive equal opportunities policies, and views such policies as a valuable contribution towards ensuring equal opportunities in employment, based solely on merit and suitability for the job'.

The statement goes on to point out that many employers who operate a formal policy of equal opportunities believe it makes sound business sense in terms of developing the full potential of their employees. It explains that it is advantageous to commit such policy to writing so that it can be made known to all the employees affected by it. (For example, by including a statement of the policy in the staff handbook.) It is important, says the CBI, for the policy to have the support of senior management, and that each company should decide for itself in the light of its own workforce composition and operational requirements the sort of policy that will be practicable for its organization. In smaller companies, the CBI says, a lesser degree of formality in the formulation and implementation of the policy might be more appropriate.

Companies should decide for themselves how best to ensure equality of opportunity, which they may wish to review from time to time, and the formality of any evaluation will vary from company to company. Those employing significant numbers of women might well find it useful to keep statistics. This might include keeping a check on whether salaries and promotion are handled in a non-discriminatory way.

The CBI urges employers to give close consideration to a number of issues arising in the field of equal opportunities such as pay, job evaluation, recruitment, training, promotion and transfer, benefits, terms of employment, discipline, redundancy and dismissal. They point out that the Codes of Practice, issued by the Equal Opportunities Commission, contain detailed guidance and recommendations on all aspects of employment for women, and, although they do not impose any legal obligations, their provisions are admissible in evidence and must be taken into account if they are relevant. In addition, the Codes of Practice contain important recommendations on the voluntary steps employers can take to promote the development of equal opportunities in employment. Such steps are frequently referred to as 'positive action'.

The CBI reminds employers that the Council of Ministers of the European Community has adopted a Recommendation for the Promotion of Positive Action for Women. Again, although not legally binding, it urges members of the European Community to assist and encourage the development of positive action for women in employment.

As the table shows, Britain lags far behind the rest of Europe when it comes to enlightened policies on women and employment, and makes no concession to the concept of parental leave — time off work for either parent following the end of maternity leave to care for the child.

Current employment conditions in the UK fail to provide adequately for the fact that women's working lives are more seriously affected than men's by having children and in caring for them. Women who do not qualify for maternity leave, who may have an unplanned pregnancy, or who do not wish to return to work immediately, will lose their continuity of employment.

Those who wish to return to work part-time (and two-thirds of women who return following a break for child-bearing do so on a part-time basis) often have to seek work in lower paid and lower status jobs, in some cases wasting valuable skills and many years' training. In 1988, the Women and Employment Survey found that as many as 45 per cent of women who had returned to work part-time after having a child, returned to a position in a lower occupational category.

Parental leave in the European Community

West Germany	10 months can be taken part-time with employers' consent. Flat rate payment for six months, then income related
France	Two years unpaid to either parent *or* right to work part-time for the same period. Flat rate payment where three or more children in the family
Italy	Six months, paid at 30 per cent of earnings
Denmark	10 weeks, paid at 90 per cent of earnings
Greece	Six months, unpaid
Portugal	Two years unpaid
Belgium	Six to twelve months, substantial leave for reasons including care of young children. Can be taken part-time. Social security

	payment when position filled by unemployed person
Luxembourg	Public sector employees, one year unpaid leave or part-time work
Ireland	Career break schemes in Civil Service
Netherlands	New scheme beginning 1988/9
Spain	Three-year career break scheme

Source: Equal Opportunities Commission.

The proposed EEC directive was published in December 1983. In 1985, a House of Lords Select Committee concluded that there should be EEC legislation for paid parental leave of one month, pointing out that such leave would help children and parents as well as promoting equal opportunity.

The concept of parental leave recognizes and encourages the role of the father in child-care, helps to achieve a more equal sharing of family responsibilities between mother and father, and allows parents to combine careers with responsible family life.

Parental leave is being established throughout the EEC as a means of promoting the welfare of children and helping parents to combine work and family commitments. Nine EEC countries already provide some form of parental leave for the whole or part of their workforce.

In the UK, fathers are currently excluded from access to any statutory leave provisions relating to the birth or care of their child, and this has led to the perpetuation of the assumption that leave arrangements for the care of young children are only necessary for mothers.

First introduced in Sweden, parental leave is now widely available in different forms throughout the European Community. Among the provisions of the proposed EEC directive are:

- A minimum of three months' leave per worker per child
- A part-time option that would effectively mean twelve months of part-time leave divided equally between mother and father instead of six months' full-time leave
- Both parents may not be on leave at the same time and leave could not be transferable

- Leave entitlement could be extended for single parents or parents of handicapped children

- An allowance may be paid to workers on leave, which would be at the discretion of each state, and would come from public funds and not from employers.

The proposals also allow for family leave to cope with important family crises, such as the serious illness of a child.

Key elements of the parental leave proposals include the option for parental child-care, the sharing of child-care between father and mother, the part-time option, flexibility.

Options for UK employers considering parental leave include:

- Converting extended maternity leave into parental leave, or offering a period of parental leave at the end of statutory maternity leave

- Allowing fathers access to part of maternity leave in place of mothers. Manchester City Council, for example, allows the father access to maternity leave in place of the mother from 12 weeks following the birth

- Separate child-care leave, as in the case of one publisher offering 20 weeks' paid child-care leave to employees.

Although parental leave is one of a number of work and family provisions, assistance with child-care flexibility in hours through job-sharing, family leave and provision for longer career breaks are all important options which employers are beginning to consider.

In spite of the emphasis on the doctrine of equal opportunities, many professions still maintain a low profile on the question of maternity leave, career breaks and provision for women working part-time.

However, a number of professions and industries that traditionally employ a large number of women are beginning to dip their toe into the waters of equal opportunities and confront the issues of maternity leave provision, career breaks and the pressures of combining work and home.

Teaching

Teaching has long been regarded as a career which a woman could ideally combine with raising her own family. However, the problem of how much maternity leave to take is left to the discretion of local authorities who are guided by the statutory rules.

The National Union of Teachers (NUT) report *Promotion and the Woman Teacher* (1980) emphasized that, although women in teaching generally take short career breaks, they are damaging women's career prospects. A Government report, based on the 1980 census also indicated that half of all women having their first baby in recent years returned to work within four years of the birth, although many initially returned to part-time work.

The NUT survey found that an estimated 65 per cent of women teachers took a break in service to bring up families. Although improved maternity provisions were introduced in 1979, this figure is still a significant percentage. One of the main recommendations of the Union's report was the need to establish more flexible patterns of promotion which recognized that the careers of women who rear families will begin later than those of their colleagues or will stop and begin again, and that these women should be judged not by their age, but by their ability.

In 1985, the NUT passed a Memorandum on Equal Opportunities in Education, which addressed itself, among other things, to the proper management of career breaks for women. This called for improved maternity and paternity leave provision by local authorities, as well as more part-time or shared posts, career counselling and training courses. In the same year, it became Union policy to protect posts and status of women taking maternity leave for one year in the school and three years in the local authority, with the right to have the same status and pay on return to a post. Some education authorities have partially agreed to these proposals. However, Kent County Council's Education Service has developed an agreement which the Union would like to see as a blueprint for others. Their agreement offers the re-employment of returners for up to seven years, as well as offering a return to the previous post or to a suitable vacancy. During the period of absence, the returner should be available for supply teaching for at least ten working days per year. In-service training is also provided during the period of leave to enable the returner to keep up to date with developments.

Various other schemes currently being considered for a more enlightened and flexible approach to women teachers leaving to have children are being carefully watched, and the NUT is keen to work towards the situation where career-break does not equal career-end for women teachers.

Doctors and the medical profession

It has reached the point where almost half of those graduating into the medical profession are women, yet only 20 per cent of family doctors are women and only 13 per cent of consultants are female, despite women comprising 25 per cent of all graduates since the 1960s.

These figures were published in a report commissioned by the Department of Health and published in June 1988, which confirmed that the outlook for women doctors is bleak, unless attitudes change. The report went on to claim that two thirds of young women doctors were so frustrated with their careers that they wished they had never gone into medicine. It also found that exhausting and stressful hours of work, disrupted or non-existent family and social life, inflexible career structures, the old-boy network and the scramble for jobs entailing moving around the country all conspired against women doctors.

The report, based on interviews with men and women who had qualified in 1966, 1976 and 1981 found that women with children and families felt excluded from top jobs. Many of the 'older' women doctors interviewed were still working, but had ended up in what were essentially 'dead end' jobs. One woman doctor summed up typical reactions to the task of combining home and medicine by saying 'It is an absolutely lousy job for a woman who wants a home, husband and family. If I had known more about the hours before I took it on, I don't think I'd have gone into it.'

If women doctors want to succeed in their profession, it would appear to be very difficult for them to develop any personal commitments or involvements, let alone marry and consider having children, for at least the first ten years of their working life. So those female doctors who have made it to senior registrar or consultant level will probably have postponed their first baby until their 30s.

Banks and financial sector

Leading the way in the financial sector are the banks, where NatWest, in particular, was among the first to make it easier for women to break their career to care for young children. They offer a period of up to five years from the date of the start of maternity leave, although the offer may be extended at the bank's discretion.

Two schemes were introduced by NatWest in 1981. The re-entry scheme is available to staff with the potential to reach senior management and who expect to return to work after having a child with their career commitment undiminished. The bank guarantees an offer of re-employment at the same level at which they left, and provides a training programme on their return, designed to update their knowledge and competence. The reservist scheme is open to staff who have the potential to reach junior/middle management and who expect to return to full-time employment. The bank does not guarantee to re-employ an individual, but will consider participants for suitable vacancies at the level at which they left.

Applicants for either scheme will normally be expected to have completed five years' service, and, on return, serve for at least another 20 years before retirement.

To keep their hand in, those on leave undertake to provide a minimum of two days' paid relief work per year (although many do more than this) and to attend an annual one-day seminar. While they are away, contact is maintained and they receive regular information packs and invitations to local social events. If appropriate, some women may continue with their studies for the Institute of Bankers examinations.

In the City of London's Square Mile financial quarter, women are increasingly taking their place in the ranks of brokers, analysts, merchant bankers, and underwriters. There are signs even here, in what must be the most traditionally male of all working environments, that employers are waking up to the fact that female employees are a valuable commodity in themselves and that child-care inducements should be offered to facilitate their return to work more easily. The first City crèche opened its doors in January 1988, followed by another in April and it looks as though more and more companies will soon be joining the bandwagon.

With world markets now open almost 24 hours a day, the working day can be very long and arduous for women at the sharp end, in capital markets, for example. For most women in this fast-moving financial sector, a live-in nanny is a must, particularly if overseas business trips are also a feature of their jobs.

One mother-to-be working in a Japanese securities firm explained that the company were very fair to women who wanted to take a break to have a baby. However, she went on to say the daily pressures of their job and the long hours meant that most women have decided it would be unrealistic to have children and expect to carry on working in international finance.

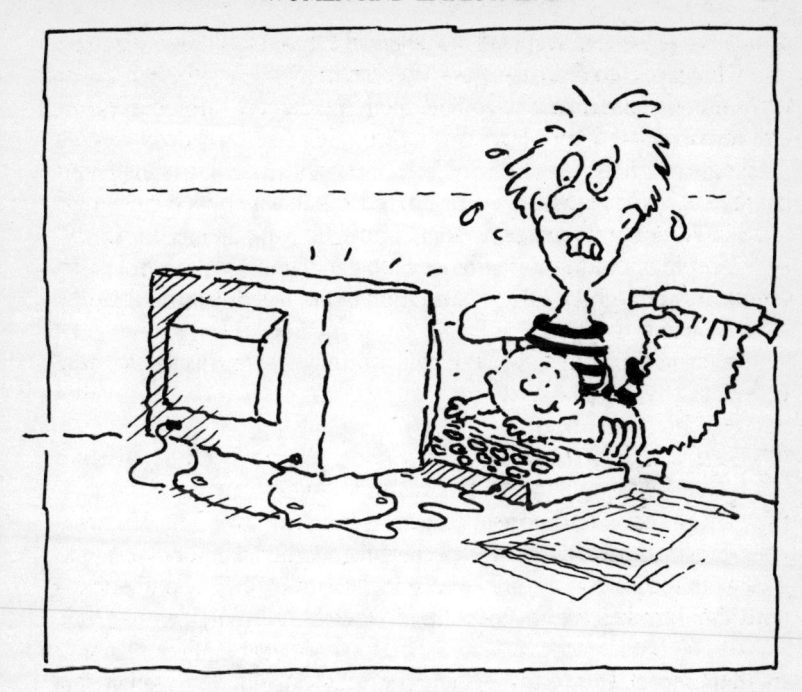

An associate director in one of the leading US merchant banks confirms that life is tough for City working mothers. Those who are trying to combine their pressured working life with being a mother were finding it an 'ongoing battle' with their emotions and their gruelling daily schedules which they manage to get through on 'autopilot' from the minute they open their eyes at the crack of dawn. A working day that stretches from seven in the morning to eight at night is not uncommon, plus the need to be away on business trips. It is very difficult to find and, more important, keep good nannies who will adapt and be understanding about the long hours they must work to cover for the mother's extended and often unpredictable working day.

Surviving this self-imposed conflict between family and a financial career call for rude good health and stamina, so it is not surprising that working mothers in senior positions are a rarity in the City. But as one of this successful species comments:

> It is very much a question of what investment you have made in your career, whether or not you will find it easy or desirable to give it all up to become a full-time mother. If you are 32 and

enjoying a high level of financial reward for what you do, and have achieved a great deal in terms of respect, status and working environment, then it becomes much more of a dilemma to turn your back on ten years' hard work.

Because it's such hard work combining the two roles, it will only make sense to continue if you really enjoy your job and are achieving a great deal of personal satisfaction and financial reward.

There is no doubt that having a baby changes your whole set of priorities and focuses your emotions in the direction of your home and children. But I really enjoy my job, otherwise I would not be here.

Public relations

The PR industry traditionally attracts a large number of women, and many of the industry's most respected and successful figures are female. However, the attitude towards maternity leave is still largely undeveloped and varies from company to company. It would seem that women who have a good track record and who have postponed their first pregnancy until their late 20s or early 30s are in a better position to negotiate their maternity leave provision, having proved their worth as an employee to clients and the firm.

Successful women executives who decide to call it a day once they become pregnant are flattered by their employer's attempts to woo them back, at least part time, so reluctant are they to lose their expertise permanently. They are then in the enviable position of being able to dictate their own terms and hours. As one woman PR executive says:

> When I realized that one of the first woman board directors to have a baby was virtually asked to resign on the spot, I did not hold out much hope for generous maternity leave provision in my own case.
>
> Although two senior board directors had taken maternity leave a couple of years earlier, both had returned very soon after the birth and resumed their full-time responsibilities.
>
> When I announced the news, I was told initially that all I could expect would be statutory maternity rights, plus a percentage of my salary for six weeks. It did not seem very generous, since I had worked hard for the firm for five years and had contributed

a great deal to its growth and expansion.

When I came out of the meeting and thought about the offer in more detail, I realized that what I wanted was only 3-4 months' leave and that, in view of what I felt was my proven worth to the company, I would try to negotiate the terms of my maternity leave. In fact, the company was then very fair and admitted that the reason why it had originally stuck more or less to statutory rights was that it had not really thought about it before. No one, except the two board directors, had ever wanted to come back to work.

Since then four other women have taken maternity leave and successfully resumed their responsibilities afterwards.

I found it quite hard work grooming someone else to take over from me while I was away and making sure that everything would run smoothly.

I did have to take a back seat for a time, too, since I was not given the promotion I would have got before I went on maternity leave, although this has now come a year later. I understood their reaction, however, as they treated me honestly and fairly and I suppose they were waiting to see if I would maintain my commitment to my career once the baby was born.

My advice to anyone asking for maternity leave would be to think logically and calmly about what you consider your worth to be and your added-value after several years' experience with the same company and present your case calmly and logically.

I did find the first few weeks of being at home with the baby quite a shock and was glad to escape for a few hours when my cleaning lady came, as I could trust her to look after the baby for a while.

The trouble is that working women don't meet full-time mothers very often and so they just do not know what to expect when they have a child of their own.

I don't know how single mothers cope on their own, with the fatigue and the constant demands of the baby.

I found that I could not even manage to clear the breakfast dishes by the end of the day in the early weeks, and wondered if I would ever manage to be able to go back to work.

I was very lucky to find an excellent nanny through the local college, and I went back to work for half days for the first two weeks and gradually built up my hours.

Although it is all working out well, I still feel tired and torn some mornings when the baby clings to me as I leave for work. I think it is probably more difficult if you have fed the baby yourself, as this increases the 'bonding' and the guilt, when you return to work.

I suppose the next trauma will be deciding when, and if, to have a second baby. One or two colleagues who were pregnant at the same time as me are already on to their second. But I still feel as if I have not recovered from the first yet, and the baby still wakes in the night and comes into our bed. We are just about to try a new attack on curing him of this... I'm not sure how successful it will be. Everyone tells me he will just stop doing it gradually.

We are also in the throes of deciding whether or not to move to the country as we need more space, but I find it comforting to live so near work. It means I can be home in 20 minutes should there be an emergency.

Publishing

Publishing is an industry staffed mainly by women. One first-time mother who works for a leading financial magazine felt that her employers were very helpful and considerate about maternity leave.

I kept getting phone calls at home to see how I was getting along and to remind me about the dates by which I should inform them officially about when I would be back.

The thing is that several other women had already been along this route and, very sensibly, the company had sorted out its position on maternity leave, so that different departments were not just doing their own thing. I was given five months' paid leave and didn't lose out on my profit share either. I felt that I had been very fairly treated.

In my case, partly because we have a small house and partly because I wanted to experience the 'sharp end of motherhood' — coping with the baby at either end of the day — I opted for a nanny share arrangement, which the NCT Nannyshare register helped me organize.

The baby is cared for from 9.30 to 6.30 by an extremely capable 27-year-old trained nanny, at the other mother's house. The children benefit from each other's company and we both feel the nanny has risen to the dual challenge magnificently. We share her £115 per week salary and her travel costs.

I was quite lucky when I was on maternity leave because my husband works freelance from home, so there were times when he was around to give me some support. Because he has had children in his first marriage, he was also able to be objective and practical in solving some of the problems. I found the lack of companionship from other mothers with whom I had anything in common quite difficult, although I was very fortunate in having an excellent health visitor who was very supportive. My parents, too, would come and spend the day and give me a break.

I was quite surprised by the way the day would drift past me in a sort of haze. I couldn't read a paper, I couldn't concentrate long enough for that. Some days I did wonder if I would ever make it back to work.

Now I am back at work and things have settled down now the baby is 14 months, apart from broken nights as a result of teething. I do find that our social life has become almost non-existent. I really do not want to go out in the evenings because I would rather be at home with the baby and dinner parties are a thing of the past.

Solicitors and barristers

It was a very early piece of anti-sex discrimination legislation in 1919, the Sex Disqualification (Removal) Act, which allowed women to enter the law in the first place. In recent years the numbers of women entering the legal profession has risen dramatically. In 1986, 44 per cent of those admitted to articles were women compared with 13 per cent in 1973 and 5 per cent in 1963. Only 37 women were admitted in 1963, compared with 1,204 in 1986. Yet, in spite of the rise in entry to the profession, the numbers of women managing to stay in the profession and reach senior levels is quite small. Only 56 per cent of women admitted in 1977 are still working full-time, and only 75 per cent of women who joined the profession in 1982 are in permanent, full-time jobs. Women generally progress much more slowly to partnership than men, and more women than men remain as assistant solicitors.

In an attempt to redress the balance in January 1988, the Law Society published a report on women's careers in the Law (*Equal in the Law*). This report highlighted the concern about the plight of women solicitors:

The picture is one where more and more women are coming into the profession, and where a significant and alarming number are temporarily retiring from it after a few years. Women have proportionately fewer practising certificates than men, reach partnership at a much slower rate than men, work part-time far more than men, and retire altogether from the profession in greater numbers. At a time when women are making up about half the current intake, and where there is a severe recruitment crisis which may last for several years, then there is clearly cause for serious concern.

It also made a number of recommendations, primarily with the intention of allowing women to be able to return to the profession after a career break. These include:

- Proposals for legislation to set different levels of practising fees. The current level of £280 per year is expensive for a woman without a separate income. The report suggests that there should be a reduced nominal level for women who are away from the profession temporarily.

- Changes in the procedures by which practising certificates are issued, so that women who have been away for a time raising children no longer have to satisfy the Law Society that they are fit to be solicitors as is the case currently. Many women find this procedure humiliating, as they have to find two solicitors who are willing to declare that they are fit to work as a solicitor, which puts them in the category of people who, in the past, have shown themselves unfit.

- The introduction of refresher courses for women coming back to the profession.

- Adopting a policy in favour of requesting tax relief for child-care expenses for women solicitors who return to work and take steps to persuade other professions and organizations to adopt this policy to increase pressure on the government to adopt it.

The report states that, since it is generally the case that the chief responsibility for looking after children rests with their mothers, and that women who wish to go out to work have to pay someone to look after the children, very often the expense and complexity of being a working mother often acts as a deterrent.

It is a very poor use of scarce taxpayers' resources to spend four years educating a person to qualify as a solicitor, allow her to practice less than ten years, and then fail to provide the tax resources to enable her to continue in that career and make available the benefits of that education for the full length of a legal career.

The report is also in favour of firms considering the advantages of part-time work, even a part-time partner, as well as viewing the career needs of women solicitors more sympathetically by becoming career-break employers. Firms are also recommended to ensure that partnership arrangements are adequate to cover for the needs of maternity leave and maternity pay of female partners.

The report comments on the prevailing attitudes that many women solicitors have had to face during their career:

> There is a prevailing attitude that children, and in some cases, marriage, will end the woman solicitor's career.
>
> I was amazed to find that I was asked all the predictable questions about child-care arrangements, my husband's attitude to my career, etc.
>
> Because I am a mother, I have been asked about my reproductive intentions at every interview . . . and cross-examined as to the arrangements for my child . . . I would prefer not to answer, but accept it would be counterproductive to refuse.

This far-reaching report is a major initiative in the promotion of equality for women in the law and is a milestone in the reconciliation of the difficulties encountered by women in fulfilling their social responsibilities for their children and families with the needs of a career.

One leading Bristol practice, at least, is already operating an enlightened part-time working scheme. The firm employs a total of 99 women out of a total staff of 130. Provided they have fulfilled two years' with the firm, the same qualification as for statutory maternity leave, they are allowed nine months off, three months longer than their statutory right. Part-time working can last until 18 months after the birth for a minimum of three days a week. All the rules apply to the birth of each successive child. In reaching its decision, the firm discovered that women generally get better class degrees than men, and that, in 1987, the number of women passing the Law Society's finals exceeded the number of men for the first time ever. However, nationally, male solicitors achieve partnerships at about twice the rate of women. The women in this practice who take advantage of its revolutionary approach feel they are among the new breed of women solicitor who will make partnership level on merit, regardless of their sex.

Accountancy

Echoes of this trailblazing approach to women in the professions are being heard in the field of accountancy, another male preserve.

The Institute of Chartered Accountants confirms that an increasing number of women are entering the profession, 35 per cent compared with only 17 per cent in 1977. As one working mother who is a partner in a leading London firm of accountants which employs a number of women says:

> It is relatively easy for a woman accountant to take time off for maternity leave. Essentially, this is because of the way accountants work, and the way in which they gear up for particular projects. It is not too difficult to say, for example, that in six months' time you will be taking six months' maternity leave. The work can very easily be moved around within the team, and people can be scheduled to take your place.
>
> What is more difficult is what happens when you come back to work and you have to reconcile the demands of children and a family life with the pressures of an essentially client-driven job, where you are expected to be available at all hours, particularly if you are in the middle of a takeover or other major corporate activity. This is when it becomes more difficult to keep some time exclusively for your family which you know you can rely on.
>
> It is easier in certain areas of accountancy, for example, tax, to be assured of more predictable hours. So perhaps women coming into the profession who also want to have a family might well be advised to look at specializations that would make it easier for them to combine their dual role.
>
> We have set up a task force to look at the whole question of women returning to work in our firm. At the end of the day, there will be limitations on what we can do because of the nature of

the profession we are in. However, among the options we looked at were job-sharing of course, and working part-time and from home, but what we really need to do is to change some of the ingrained attitudes we keep coming up against.

It is not so difficult with the people who work for the firm, since the younger generation of men would also welcome a more understanding attitude towards family responsibilities and the need to spend time with their wife and children. Ironically, it is often among the clients that we encounter the most resistance and an unwillingness to be flexible. You are simply expected to be available when needed, and that's that.

On balance, a woman considering combining a career in accountancy with a family and children will need to have tremendous stamina and a co-operative and flexible partner who will support her at home and shoulder equal responsibilities for child-care and the domestic arrangements whenever she is preoccupied at work. That is why it is advisable to get your professional qualifications under your belt before embarking on motherhood as it will be very difficult to study and work while you have young children.

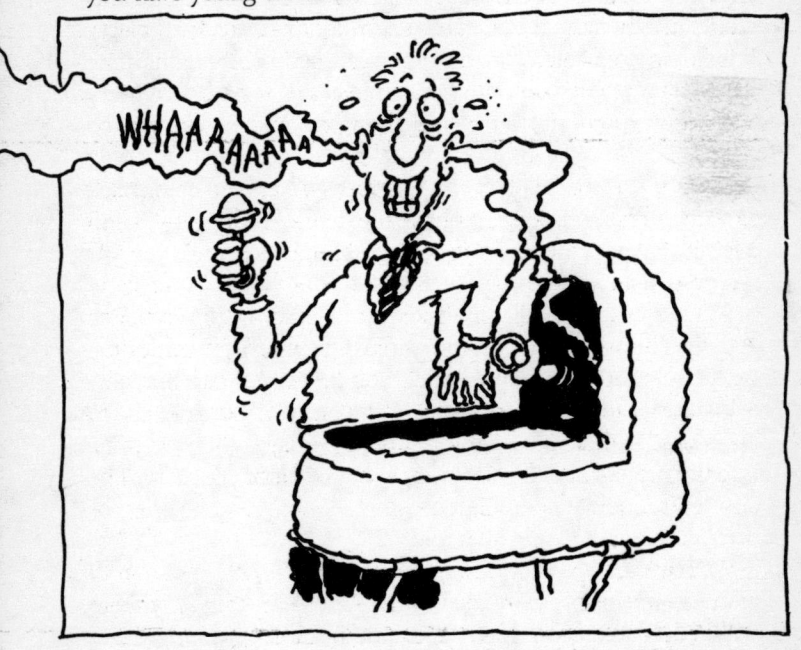

In looking at these various careers and professions, one begins to see that there is a common denominator for all working mothers. Stamina is essential to their survival, backed up by good health, a supportive husband or partner and, ideally, a sympathetic employer and working environment.

Every second counts for these women who need to run their lives like clockwork in order to keep everything running smoothly the whole time. If one cog of their well-oiled domestic machine stops turning, then the whole delicately balanced daily mechanism could break down, except that, in most cases, it doesn't because of one vital component on permanent 24-hour standby — the woman of the house — who will be expected to perform the usual miracle and avert yet another crisis of conflict between family and career.

CHAPTER SIX
Finance and a family

When you become a mother, you will join the ranks of the ultimate consumer, and become a prime target for the £10 million or so spent annually on advertising baby equipment, clothes, food, nappies and skin-care products. In short, you will number among those who are helping the manufacturers of 'slings and buggies to make outrageous fortunes'. And it does not just stop at advertising in the media.

If you annouce the birth of your baby in the columns of a national newspaper (and that in itself will set you back a few pounds), naming the hospital where the delivery took place, instead of the avalanche of greetings cards from long-lost schoolfriends who you hoped would see your name, you are more likely to be deluged by sales literature from life insurance companies and banks encouraging you to take out school fees policies, children's accident cover, and open savings accounts.

From the moment you suspect you are pregnant, and perhaps even before, if you are the sort to buy books and magazines on a new topic of interest, your hand will never be out of your pocket. Having a baby in style will cost you a lot of money. And you will wonder what on earth you ever found to spend your double income on before. The baby-boom-driven market is rapidly expanding and becoming so diverse that you are likely to fall prey to its temptations even before you are pregnant.

Your first foray might well result in the purchase of one of the new cycle predictors which claim to help you pinpoint the best time for conception to take place. If all goes well, and you suspect you are pregnant, you may then be tempted to buy a home pregnancy testing kit. Gone are the romantic announcements over a candle-lit dinner with your unsuspecting, shocked husband. He will probably be acting as laboratory assistant, timing the test with deadly precision in your bathroom at the crack of dawn on the appointed day.

From then on it is onwards and upwards to the cosmetic counter for

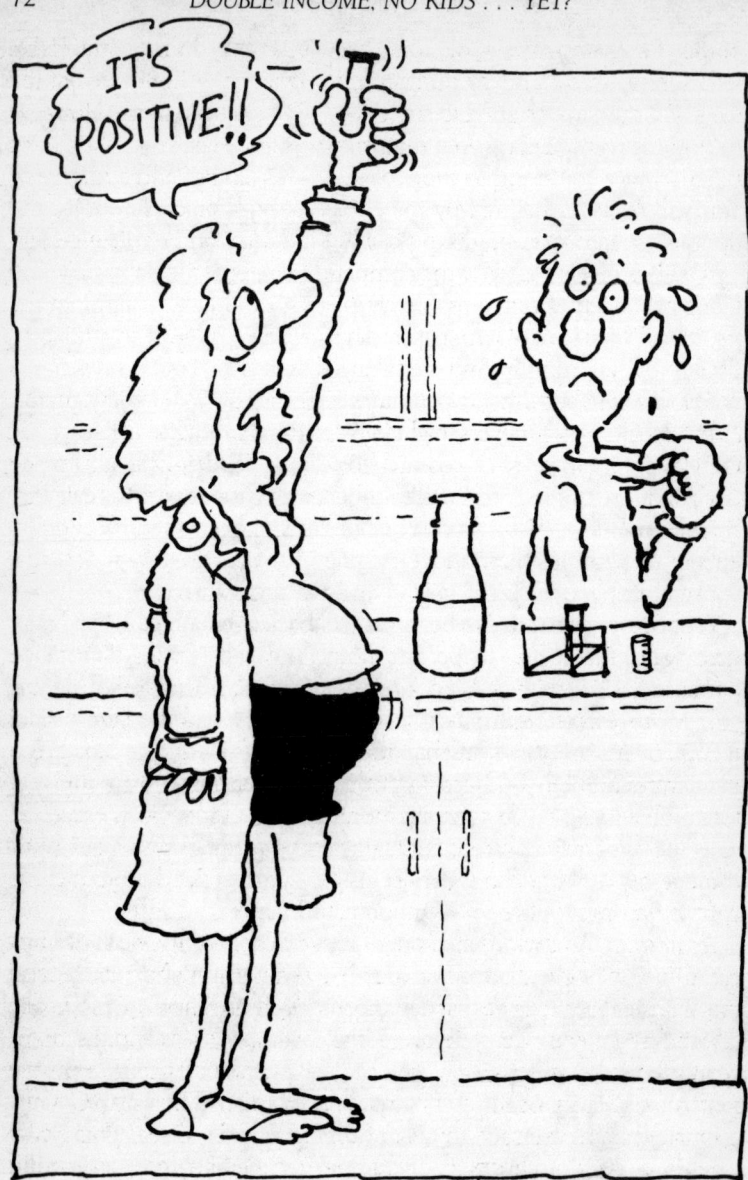

the best in anti-stretch mark creams, or extra vitamins or fluoride tablets. Once your expanding waistline can no longer be contained by your pre-pregnancy clothes, you will be seduced by the wide and imaginative range of designer maternity clothes, enlarging your wardrobe to include outfits for every aspect of your hectic lifestyle, from comfortable voluminous track suits or dungarees for relaxing at home to tailored suits and dresses designed to streamline your shape at work. However, the fortune you spend on your maternity wardrobe will seem like a mere pittance once you begin to shop for the baby's clothes and equipment. You will be overwhelmed by the choice of both practical outfits and designer clothes, cots, prams, pushchairs, car seats, and sterilizing units. You will be mesmerized by the competing claims of the baby milk and foods producers and disposable nappy brigade, unless you opt for the traditional, high quality, terry nappy. That in itself will mean an additional weekly bill for laundry and sterilizing powders.

To follow will be further expenditure on high chairs, stair safety guards, electric socket safety covers, night lights, baby alarms, and car seats, not to mention books, toys, videos and story tapes. So rapidly is this market developing, with new products being launched almost every week, that by the time you have a second baby you will be made to feel guilty for not owning the latest and 'even safer' baby buggy, or car seat that you will feel you ought to go out and buy it all again.

Your nursery will need to be furnished, decorated and equipped and, here again, the costs can be astronomical if you opt for handmade furniture, designer blinds and curtains, stencilling, borders, with matching crib, Moses basket and cot. In fact, you could spend the best part of £2,000 on essential equipment and clothing in the first year alone. You may even find that you need to move to a larger house, or, at the very least, substitute the Porsche for a more sedate and capacious estate car. This will probably be more damaging for your image than your bank balance, but is very often the most visible sign that the double-income couple has come of age and become a family.

Apart from the obvious spending-spree that heralds the birth of a first child, you may decide to have your baby in a private hospital — and this is one delivery charge that does not come cheap. There are essentially two main elements of cost involved: the consultant's fees and the 'hotel' costs for your post-natal stay in a private room at a specialist private maternity hospital or in the private wing of an NHS hospital. Overall, estimates put the average total cost of ante-natal and post-natal maternity care in a London hospital, including consultant's fees, at around £2,000-£2,500. Outside London, this could fall to around £1,600-£1,800. You should expect to pay between £200-£300 per night for accommodation, for an average stay of about 7-8 days for a first baby, and longer if you have a Caesarean, or if there are complications.

Consultant's fees will cost between £800-£1,000, and the anaesthetist, if you need an epidural injection or have a Caesarean, will charge about £175-£200.

That is not all. You should expect to pay for absolutely every item you use, from the smallest cotton bud to dressings and safety pins. You will also have to pay the costs of any pre-natal tests such as ultrasound, or any X-rays or pathology tests you may need.

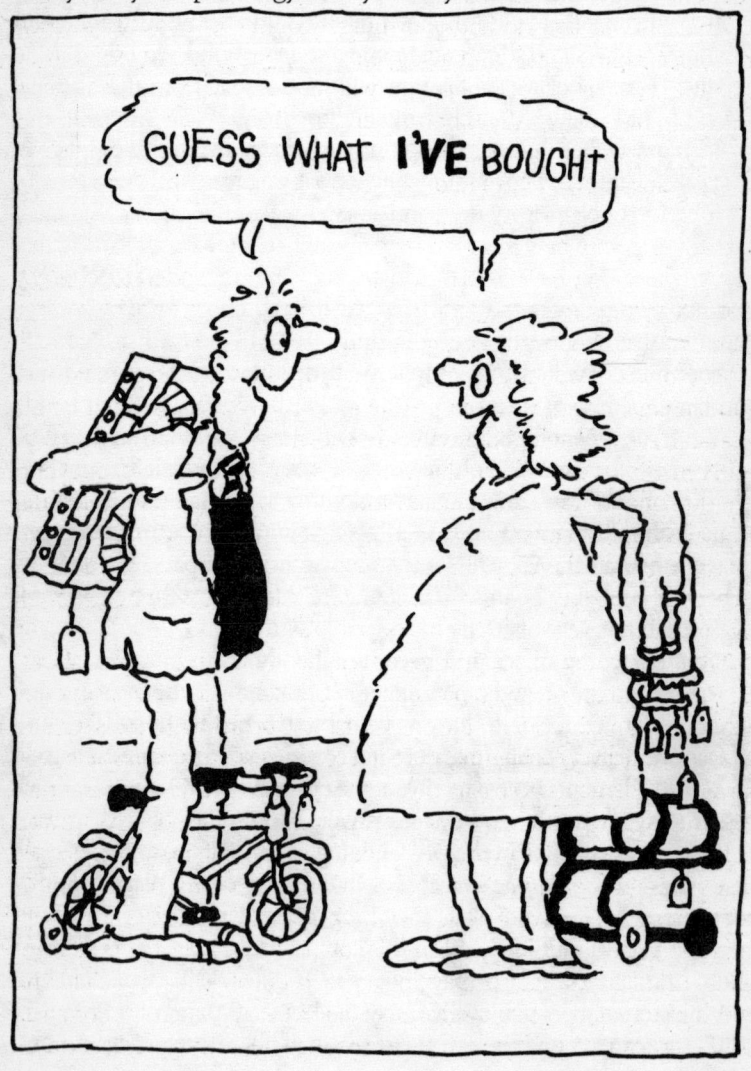

When you return from hospital, irrespective of whether or not you are planning to have a live-in nanny when you go back to work, you might want to engage the assistance of an experienced maternity nurse for the first six weeks to help you to settle the baby into a routine and give you a bit of support to catch up on sleep, share night feeds and so on. You will find this especially important if you are planning to return to work sooner rather than later.

An ad in *The Lady* to find your nurse would cost about £50 (and, of course, you may not find a suitable applicant). Agency fees start at about £120. Her salary, which you will have to pay from the day she moves in before the baby is born, even if the baby is late, will be in the region of £35 per day (£245 per week) plus board and lodgings.

On-going, longer term child-care costs are covered in Chapter 4.

Education

Once you pass out of the baby and toddler stage, your thoughts will start to dwell on education, and, here again, you will need to make the fundamental choice between private and state education. Such is the pressure even on the good private nursery schools, let alone on the prep and boarding school places, that you will be advised to at least put your child's name down at birth. Even the £20-£30 registration fees for a nursery school place when your child is three years old can mount up, as you may need to put your name down at two or three schools since you will probably be told you will have to go onto a waiting list even at that early stage.

The average cost of private education now runs from about £1,800-£3,000 per year for a preparatory day school to the upper range of nearly £2,000 per term for one of the top boarding schools. On to that you have to add uniforms and extra activities such as piano or tennis lessons. Many couples facing this sort of expense will be reluctant to lose the woman's salary if this means having to forfeit the option of private schools altogether. For while the childless double-income couple are able to regard the woman's earnings as a bonus, enabling them to enjoy a high standard of living, once they have a family, this salary may well become a necessity if they are to maintain their lifestyle *and* be able to afford the highest standards of child-care and education for their children.

A high earner gives up more than her job and salary when she becomes a full-time mother and she can also lose much of her independent existence outside the home. It also means having to adjust to reduced budgets and a more economical way of life, and financial dependence on her husband, which, when it happens, may be less attractive than it seemed.

Tax reform for women

The rise in the numbers of working women with financial independence was finally officially recognized by the government in the April 1988 Budget. Sweeping reforms for married couples were introduced, giving married women independent financial status in relation to their personal income and capital tax allowance. From April 1990, married women will be recognized as people in their own right by the taxman. From that date, married women will pay their own tax, on the basis of their own income, and fill in their own tax return when one is necessary.

When the reforms are introduced, a married woman will get the same personal allowance as her husband. The husband will also get a married couple's allowance which can be transferred to his wife if he does not earn enough to use it all.

The reforms also extend to capital taxation, whereby a woman may also have her own capital gains tax allowance, whereas previously she had to share one allowance with her husband. This means that a woman can now conduct her financial affairs with complete privacy, if she so wishes.

One of the most significant elements of this Budget was the abolition of double allowances on mortgage tax relief for single people living together and sharing a mortgage. From August 1988, this arrangement was discontinued with mortgage tax relief being limited to £30,000 per property, irrespective of the number of borrowers. (Mortgages arranged before that date will continue as before.)

This reform of the mortgage relief tax provision to one per property signalled the end of the benefit of a dual allowance for single people living together and sharing the mortgage. Before August 1988, the financial implications of deciding to get married because a couple wanted to have a family were quite significant, since by following tradition, they would be worse off financially than a double-income couple who were living together. The Chancellor admitted that his Budget was designed to 'eliminate, for all practical purposes, all the tax penalties, which under the present system, can arise on marriage'. He did this because the Government was concerned that the dual tax benefit was acting as a disincentive for couples to get married and, consequently, undermining the supremacy of the family in society. Another anomaly that existed under the previous system was that unmarried couples with children could each claim the additional personal allowance intended for single parents, thus getting more tax relief than a married couple in the same position. From April 1989, they will be confined to a single additional personal allowance. However, whatever the rules and regulations about taxation, personal allowances and the like, having a baby will put a strain on your income. If a woman gives up her job to look after the baby herself, she will not only risk losing her salary in the medium-term while she takes a career break of whatever length, she may seriously damage her long-term career prospects and her lifetime earnings potential. If a woman returns to work soon after her baby is born, she will pay a high price in terms of child-care costs, which will represent a considerable proportion of her salary.

However you approach the dilemma of having and caring for children, there will be considerable financial disadvantages. The question is which you consider to be more rewarding and more important, and what price you are prepared to pay, or what sacrifices you are prepared to make, for a family life and children.

CHAPTER SEVEN
A word on behalf of fathers

'Behind every successful man you will find a strong woman', or so the saying goes. But nowadays, it is quite likely that you could put it the other way round. The increase in double-income, twin career marriages means that very often it is the woman who needs the support and understanding of a sympathetic partner if she is to be able to balance the demands and pressures of home, children and a full-time job. Perhaps in society's anxiety about allowing women to break out of the domestic mould to compete on equal terms with men at work, we overlook the implications of this major change of direction for women on the men in their life.

Just as a new breed of independent, working woman has emerged in the late twentieth century, so too has the role of men, husbands and fathers been transformed in the wake. Many men may still be uneasy at the compromises they are being asked to make within the new structure of partnerships and marriage where the emphasis is much more on a sharing of the roles. The inclusion of the term 'couplehood' in a Dictionary of New Words (*Longman Guardian New Words*) reflects the equality in partnerships which characterize the modern relationship between men and women.

Only 8 per cent of men live in the 'traditional' marriage, where father is the sole breadwinner and mother stays at home to look after an average of 2 children. With a growing number of women earning a salary and having financial independence, one of the traditional links which tied a woman to her husband has been weakened. Many women do not necessarily need their husband to provide material security in their lives. A new set of rules has been drawn up in which the focus is much more on the strength of the relationship itself, with the accent on mutuality and sharing, rather than on the 'pipe and slippers' approach where the wife essentially ran the home to fit in with the father's routines and needs.

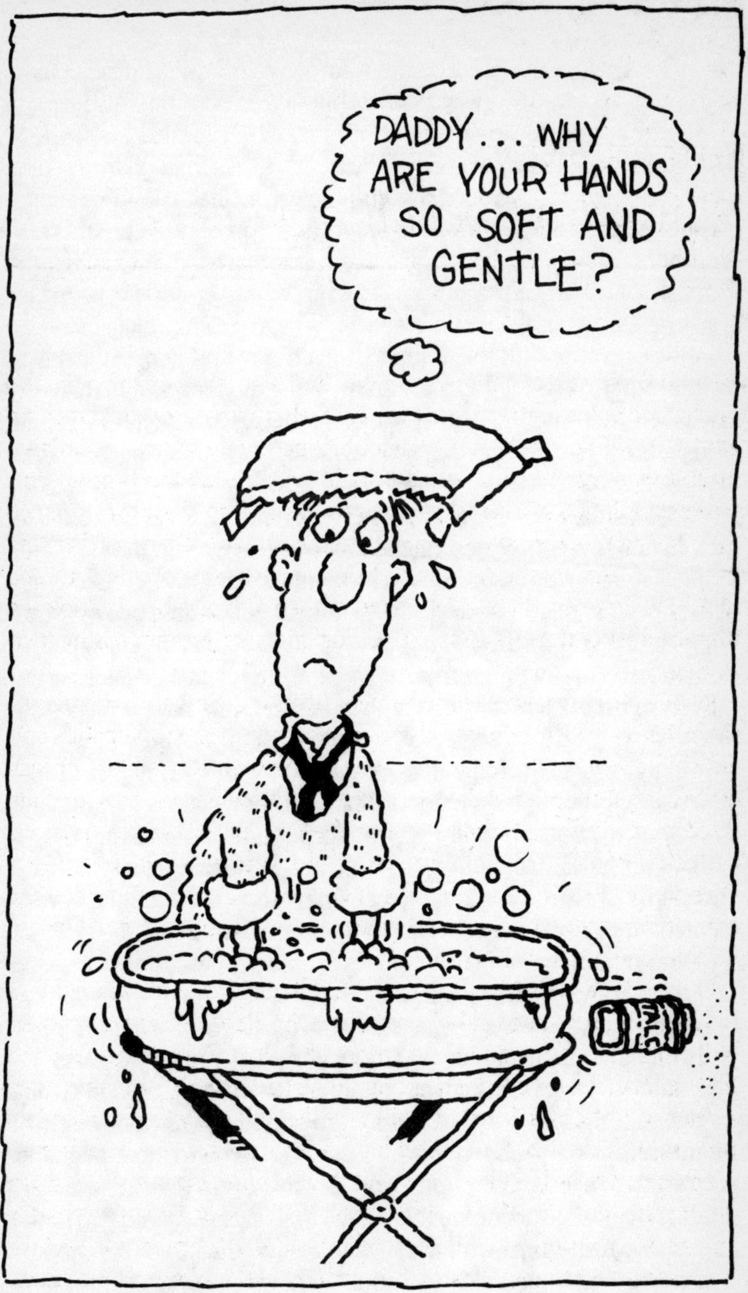
DADDY . . . WHY ARE YOUR HANDS SO SOFT AND GENTLE?

Men are now used to having to ring their working wife's secretary to leave a message and to take their turn for her to return their call. It used to be the wife who always complained that her husband was a 'workaholic', that he never came home, that he regarded his work as his only source of identity, and that he could not get through the evening or weekend without making a telephone call to the States. These days it could just as easily be the wife or girlfriend preoccupied in this way with her busy job, while her male partner is expected to shoulder the domestic burdens until she surfaces from whatever crisis is taking up her time. However, women are generally more adept at juggling their priorities at work with the demands of a home and family. Once you have children, it will fall to the woman to set the tone and manage the household along with her other responsibilities. No matter how helpful a husband or partner may be, his is essentially a supporting role, partly because most men do not know enough about it to be able to take the leading role in child-care. This is where the tensions arise, for no matter how liberated a couple you might have been, once you have children it is the woman who assumes overall care of the baby, and, consequently, of the home. While she may do this naturally, you should be aware that, at times, she will resent that it is always she who has to reorganize *her* schedule to cope with a crisis, or to be at the child's bedside during the night, no matter how early a meeting she may have arranged the next morning. So long as you can meet her half-way, you will go some part of the way to avoiding major conflict in your own relationship. If you can help her, at least emotionally, with the burdens of family life, then your relationship will become deeper and more rewarding.

However, let us spare a thought for the modern male/father/husband, forced to adapt to the implications of living with today's working woman. Denied the right of his Victorian forerunner to remain aloof and withdrawn from the mundane routines of domestic and family life, except to intervene and exercise the head of the household veto when it suited him, he is now expected to take an active part in running the home and bringing up the children. The rise in dual career marriages has introduced a new dimension into family and domestic life. On the whole, men accept that they should share in the domestic responsibilities. It is quite acceptable to be seen pushing the trolley around the supermarket each week, to help with the housework or cook dinner. The trend towards couples living together rather than marrying has encouraged this notion of equal partnership, with each member of the team contributing financially and practically to running things. But while this equal partnership and sharing of responsibilities may work quite well when there are just the two of you, what about the effects on your arrangements if you decide to have a baby?

Here again, men are expected to become actively involved in their wife's pregnancy and labour. Their fathers were allowed no further than the front door of the maternity wing, and would have run a mile if the doors of the labour ward had been opened to them, preferring the solitude and dignity of the corridor.

Nowadays, fathers' night at the ante-natal class and tours around the hospital are all designed to involve him in the momentous event. He is expected to bath a lifelike doll during the practical bath demonstration, and is taught how to spray his wife with mineral water at appropriate moments during labour, to remind her of her breathing techniques, and work with her in an active birth, sometimes even literally to support her. Most capitulate, albeit reluctantly, and one cannot help but feel rather sorry for them, as they seem to be permanently in the way in the labour ward.

In spite of your efforts, you will probably only succeed in irritating your wife by having a detailed technical discussion with the nurses about the merits of different computers and monitoring equipment while she is in the middle of a painful contraction, but at the end of the day she will be glad you are there, at what must be 'for better or worse' in its rawest form, where a torrent of verbal abuse may well be your only thanks as labour intensifies.

Your reward for your participation in this endurance test will be the right to regale the entire office with the graphic details of your wife's labour as you hand round the cigars and champagne, and a sense of pride and achievement that 'you were there the whole time'.

Ironically, you will be allowed this moment of glory with your colleagues while your wife is more likely to slip quietly back to her desk without any fuss, lest it be taken as a sign that by talking about her baby she has lost interest in her job. Colleagues may enquire, out of politeness, 'What did you have, dear?' as though it were some dreadful disease, best not talked about.

However, immediately after the baby is born, no matter how much you are encouraged to be involved, it will be your wife and the new baby who are joint top-of-the-bill and you will be called on to play the supporting role quietly in the background. A new baby is very much its mother's responsibility and you may feel a bit left out in the early weeks and months. Just like motherhood, the role of the first-time father takes time to develop and you should be patient because your time will come.

On the other hand, you may feel quite grateful that you can drift back to sleep when the baby needs attention in the night, confident that there is nothing you could do anyway, and without the slightest tinge of guilt. The best contribution you can make at this time is to support your wife emotionally and to oil the domestic wheels as much as possible.

During her pregnancy, you will have seen your wife or partner transformed from an active, dynamic, organized and energetic individual into a sleepy, vague, often forgetful creature, who retires to her bed as soon as she returns from the office surrounded by iron pills, books on pregnancy and breathing techniques, ante-natal exercises and child-care.

You will probably heave a sigh of relief once the baby arrives thinking that life will get back to normal. Don't you believe it. Things will get much worse before they get better and 'normality', as you knew it before having a family will never return again. If you decide to have a live-in nanny, you will need to take on another new persona of 'domestic employer' and all that that entails.

You will probably become impatient and irritated by your wife who, you will no doubt feel, is taking rather a long time to pull herself together. 'But you have been at home all day', you will say, as you return to an unmade bed, disorganized kitchen and no dinner for the third night running, little realizing how preoccupied she will have been all day with the baby.

It is difficult for a man to appreciate the powerful impact of the hormonal and emotional changes that happen to women in late pregnancy and the early months after the birth.

If your wife is unfortunate enough to suffer from a more lasting form of post-natal depression which may need medical intervention, then, more than ever, she will need your full support and patience.

And even when your own personal 'Mary Poppins' — calm and competent — arrives to take over, you will probably be cast in the role of confessor/counsellor by being forced to listen to your wife's concern as to whether she has chosen the right person; is she doing the right thing going back to work so soon, and so on.

You may wish at times you could return to the carefree days of being able to go out exactly when you wished. The most liberated, independent, strong-minded, confident woman can become anxious, over-emotional and, you may feel, overprotective to the baby. But this is quite normal and you should try to support and understand her as much as possible in the first few weeks, and not pressurize her into being superwoman. You will have to accept that elegant dinner parties, or even casual suppers with friends will disappear from your social calendar for a while — unless you do the cooking.

The new mother will be at her most vulnerable when she first goes back to work, and there will be times she will confide to you that she feels like giving it all up and staying at home. If you suspect this is just in reponse to pressure and problems, remind her of her long-term goals and objectives and try to help her to be more objective about whatever problems are being experienced. Remind her of her ambitions which may have become obliterated in the post-natal mists which can surround her for the first two or three months.

It may be even more difficult for the father if he feels that a woman should give up her job to stay at home and be a full-time mother. If you insist that she does and she finds she is bored and resentful, you could be responsible for a serious deterioration in your relationship.

It is often more difficult for a father who has been married before to be as excited about the birth of this child as the second wife who is having *her* first baby. It is important, for example, to be aware of the possibility that she might be disappointed in herself, albeit unnecessarily, for having produced you another daughter when you already have two by your first wife. In spite of a new-found independence, natural and traditional female reactions will rear up at times of pregnancy and childbirth, in even the most liberated of women.

In general, you will have to adjust to a realignment of your life. A mother will focus her energies on her new baby and, particularly if she works, she will want to spend as much time as possible with her child when she is at home. Be selective in your social life so that you do not waste valuable time that could be spent with the child. You will find a new centre of balance, a pivot around which to base your extended relationship.

The birth of a baby to a couple who have been used to a double-income lifestyle and all the freedom and flexibility this entails, will call for just as much adjustment for the man as for the woman. And if, secretly, you are a traditionalist at heart and have always felt somewhat emasculated and uneasy about having an independent wife with a well-defined existence outside your marriage or relationship, this will be an opportunity to display some of the attitudes of support and caring associated with the traditional marriage of long ago. And for once, your wife will probably not object to your taking on the mantle of the protective mate!

References and further information

Maternity pay and employment rights

The DHSS publishes two publications which give details of your employment rights and benefits when you have a baby. These can be obtained free through your local DHSS office. They are:

Maternity Benefits: A guide to Statutory Maternity Pay, Maternity Allowance and Social Fund Maternity Payments

Babies and benefits: A guide for expectant and new mothers

The checklist and timetable which appears on pages 88-89 shows what you must do to ensure you get all your benefit and when to inform employers that you intend to give up work and when you plan to return.

Finding a nanny, mother's help or other child-care

There are three main ways of finding your first nanny. (By the time you are looking for a second nanny, you will also be able to use your contacts with nannies you have met through your own nanny to find someone who is looking for a new job.) The three ways are:

- Advertise in one of the 'nanny' magazines such as *The Lady* or *Nursery World*.

- Contact the NNEB or NAMCW Course Tutor at your local further education college and send her details of your requirements if you want a newly qualified nanny. Newly qualified nannies are usually available from the end of their final term in June.

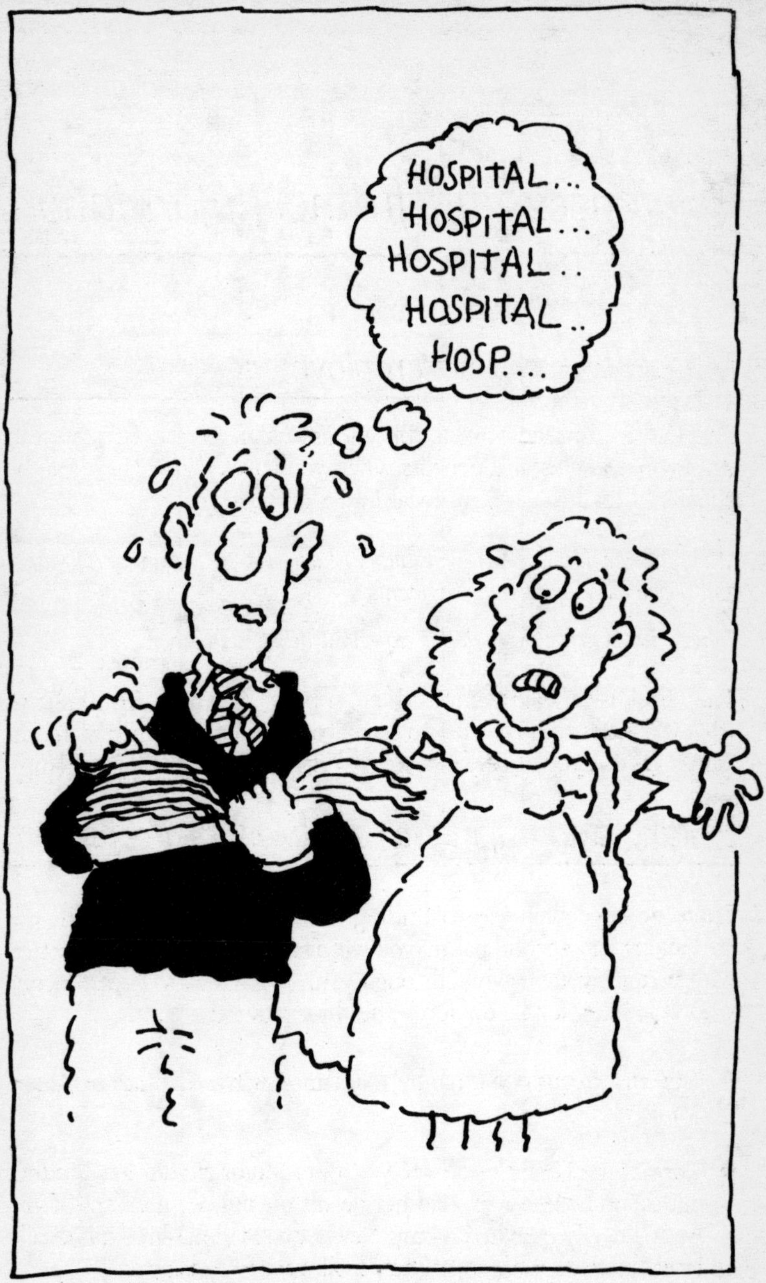
HOSPITAL...
HOSPITAL...
HOSPITAL...
HOSPITAL...
HOSP....

When	What to do	Why
As soon as you know you are pregnant	1 Ask GP or midwife for Form FW8. 2 Tell dentist (if you need treatment). 3 Check leaflets MV11, H11 and G11, tell Social Security office or FIS Unit if getting Supplementary Benefit or FIS. 4 If you are working, tell your employer. 5 Find out if you can get Maternity Allowance.	1 To apply for free prescriptions. 2 To apply for free treatment. 3 To check right to vouchers for glasses, free milk and vitamins, help with hospital fares and Social Fund Maternity Payment. 4 To find out if you can get SMP and to make sure you don't lose pay for keeping antenatal appointments. 5 If you can't get SMP.
3 weeks before you stop work	Tell your employer in writing that you will be stopping work, the week the baby is due, and if you intend to return to your job.	To protect your right to SMP and return to work.
After 26 weeks pregnant	1 Ask your doctor or midwife for a maternity certificate (form Mat BI) showing when your baby is due. 2 If you are employed, give Mat BI to your employer. 3 If you cannot get SMP, ask at your antenatal clinic or Social Security office for form MA1. 4 If your baby is due before 6 April 1987, check Maternity Grant on page 5.	1 You will need this to get either SMP or Maternity Allowance. 2 To protect your right to SMP and allow your employer to work out your entitlement. If you delay later than 3 weeks after your SMP could have started, you may lose your SMP. 3 You can apply now for Maternity Allowance on form MA1 if you cannot get SMP. 4 You may be able to get Maternity Grant.
After 29 weeks pregnant	1 If your baby is due on or after 6 April 1987 apply for a Social Fund Maternity Payment if you are getting Supplementary Benefit or FIS.	1 To pay for things for the baby.
After 34 weeks pregnant	1 If you wish to get the full 18 weeks SMP or Maternity Allowance you should stop work by the end of this week. 2 If your baby is due before 6 April 1987 check lump sum payments.	1 You may lose part of your SMP or Maternity Allowance if you work longer. 2 You may be able to get a lump sum payment.

When	What to do	Why
As soon after the birth as you can	1 Register the baby's birth. 2 Send off application form for Child Benefit (and One Parent Benefit). 3 Check low income benefits. 4 If baby was born before 6 April 1987 check Maternity Grant on page 5.	1 To get a birth certificate and NHS card. 2 To get Child Benefit (and One Parent Benefit). 3 To see if an extra child qualifies you for Supplementary Benefit, FIS, prescriptions, dental treatment, vouchers for glasses. 4 You may be able to get Maternity Grant.
By 6 weeks after birth (3 weeks in Scotland)	Register the baby's birth.	This is the latest date you can do it.
7 weeks after the week in which the baby was due	Reply in writing within 2 weeks to any letter from your employer asking if you are going back to work.	To protect your right to return to work.
3 weeks before returning to work	Write to employer that you wish to return.	To protect your right to return to work.
3 months after the birth	1 If your baby was born before 6 April 1987 you should have applied for Maternity Grant. 2 If your baby was born on or after 6 April 1987 and you or your partner are getting Supplementary Benefit or FIS apply for a Social Fund Maternity Payment if you haven't already done so.	1 You may lose maternity grant if you haven't claimed it by now. You will lose the grant if you claim more than 12 months after the birth. 2 You will lose a Social Fund Maternity Payment if you haven't claimed it by now.
29 weeks from the beginning of the week of the birth	Latest time by which you have a right to go back to your job.	You may lose your right to return.
As soon as you need them	If you get Supplementary Benefit, write to Social Security office listing things you need for older baby.	You may get lump sum payments for things like a push chair, high chair or safety gates.

Source: Reproduced from DHSS booklet, *Babies and Benefits Leaflet FB8* (HMSO, 1987).

- Register your vacancy with a local nanny agency. Addresses and telephone numbers can be obtained from your local Yellow Pages or they may advertise their services in *The Lady*. Be prepared for a hefty fee.

Try to talk to the girls on the telephone before arranging a personal interview. Talk to as many girls as you can to try and build up a picture of the sort of person you want. This is particularly important when choosing a nanny for the first time. If they show more interest in their time off or whether they can have boyfriends to visit than in the baby itself, be on your guard. I chose my first nanny because she was the only one of 10 who applied who asked what the baby's current routines were. And she proved an excellent choice.

Don't forget to ask them about their own family life. Very often this will have a strong influence on the way they behave towards the baby and, indeed, towards you, and on how they integrate into your household.

It is also advisable to draw up a list or contract outlining duties, time off, etc. A lot of problems are caused simply by misunderstanding on both sides.

The most widely read magazine by job-seeking nannies and mother's help is:

The Lady magazine
39–40 Bedford Street
London WC2E 9ER Tel: 01-379 4717

Copy must be submitted in writing. Ads received by first post on Wednesday will appear the following week.

Nanny share

Rather than employing a residential full-time nanny, you may want to organize a nanny-share, whereby your child will be cared for by a professional nanny at your home or the home of the other child, or alternately at each home, whatever you agree between yourselves.

You could begin by contacting:

NCT Nanny Share Register
Alexander House
Oldham Terrace, Acton
London W3 Tel: 01-992 8637

The NCT is a useful source of names and addresses of mothers in your area interested in nanny share arrangements. You could also try advertising in the local post office, newsagent or clinic. Some babywear shops offer a noticeboard service for such ads.

Childminder

Another much used option by working mothers is to take the child to the home of a registered childminder. Childminders care for a small number of children in their own home. They are restricted as to the number of babies and young children at one time. You can get a list of names and addresses from the Social Services Department of your local council. You could also contact:

The National Childminding Association
8 Masons Hill
Bromley
Kent BR2 9EU Tel: 01-464 6164

Nursery or workplace crèche

You may want to try to find a crèche for your child at or near your place of work. These are becoming more popular and one or two professional child-care organizations are running them on behalf of companies who provide subsidized places for employees' children. Fathers have just as much right to apply for a place for their child as the mother.

Some useful contacts are:

Workplace Nurseries Campaign
Room 205
Southbank House
Black Prince Road
London SE1 7SJ Tel: 01-582 7199

National Childcare Campaign
Wesley House
4 Wild Court
London WC2B 5AU Tel: 01-405 5617

City Child Day Nursery
1 Bridgewater Square
London EC2 Tel: 01-374 0939

The City Child Day Nursery organizes workplace crèches and has set up a successful City creche in an American Merchant Bank.

Support groups for working mothers

The National Childbirth Trust (NCT)
Alexander House
Oldham Terrace, Acton
London W3 Tel: 01-992 8637

The NCT offers all kinds of support, including antenatal classes and preparation for labour and childbirth, support in the post-natal period and advice on breastfeeding, etc., contact with working mothers groups and nanny share registers. You will be put in touch with your local group. One specialist group has developed out of the NCT:

The Working Mothers Association
248 Lavender Hill
Battersea
London SW11 1BA Tel: 01-228 3757

Meetings are held in the evenings and at weekends.

Support and advice is also given to working mothers by:

The Women Returners' Network
Ann Bell,
Secretary WRN
c/o Chelmsford AEI
Patching Hall Lane
Chelmsford
Essex CM1 4DB

If you are a single parent there are two organizations which can offer specific help and put you in touch with others in the same situation:

Gingerbread
35 Wellington Street
London WC2E MBN Tel: 01-240 0953

National Council for One Parent Families
255 Kentish Town Road
London NW5 2LX Tel: 01-267 1361

National organizations campaigning for women's rights

Equal Opportunities Commission
Overseas House
Quay Street
Manchester M33 3HN Tel: 061-833 9244

Chairwoman: Joanna Foster
Head of Policy Unit: Bronwen Cohen

This organization campaigns on behalf of equal rights for women in employment. Bronwen Cohen's address to the Industrial Society Conference in March 1988 (quoted in Chapter 1) highlighted the way the UK lags behind Europe in parental leave and pointed out the damaging impact of childbearing on a woman's potential lifetime earnings.

The EOC publishes a number of useful publications, listed below. The others listed may be obtained from the organizations in brackets.

Equal Opportunities: A Guide for Employers
A Short Guide to the Sex Discrimination Act 1975
Equal Pay: A Guide to the Equal Pay Act (Department of Employment)
Equal Pay for Work of Equal Value: A Practical Guide to the Law (CBI)
Equal Pay for Work of Equal Value: A Guide to the Amended Equal Pay Act
Job Evaluation Schemes Free of Sex Bias

Relevant legislation includes:

Sex Discrimination Act, 1975
Equal Pay (Amendment) Regulations, 1983
EOC Code of Practice for the elimination of racial discrimination and the promotion of equality of opportunity in employment
EEC Directive on Equal Pay for Men and Women (75/117/EEC of February, 1975)
EEC Directive on Equal Treatment for Men and Women (76/207/EEC of February, 1976)
EEC Recommendation on the promotion of Positive Action for Women (December, 1984)

Women's National Commission advises government on specific issues of interest to women and produces reports. (See Stress report below.)

Women's National Commission
Government Offices
Great George Street
London SW1P 3AQ
Tel: 01-270 5902

Reports on women and employment

Lifestyle and trends analysis:
Women 2000
Mintel Publications Ltd.
KAE House
7 Arundel Street
London WC2R 3DR Tel: 01-386 1814 or 01-379 3536
Price £550 (March, 1988)

Examines the new look for women in 21st century and the changing pattern of work and employment for women.

CBI Statement on Equal Opportunities Policy

CBI Statement and Guide on the principles of equal opportunities in employment.

Commends employers to consider and implement the recommendations in the CBI Statement and Guide prepared by the Equal Rights Panel which they based on members' practical experience of operating such policies in their own companies. The CBI states that its Guide is intended to be 'no more than an indication of the general principles and practice so that member companies may assess their own policy on equal opportunities and take appropriate action'.

Available from the CBI
Centre Point
103 New Oxford Street
London WC1 Tel: 01-379 7400

Index

abortion, 22
accountants, women, 69
adoption, supply of babies, 24
adoption, working mothers, 23, 24
age, maternal, 9, 10, 14, 20, 21-22, 23, 24
ambition and motherhood, 10
amnesia, maternal, 32
amniocentesis, 22
artificial insemination, 23
au pairs, child-care, 45-46

baby blues, 31
baby bug, 17
banks, women in, 61
barristers, women, 67
best time to have a baby, 17-26
  best for baby, 22-23
  biologically, 19-20
  career implications, 25
biological time clock, 9
blood pressure, 22

career break, 10, 54
career conflict, 10
career choices and pregnancy, 25, 26
career — motherhood dilemma, 7, 9
careers and working mothers, 59-70
  accountancy, 68
  banking and finance, 59
  doctors, medical, 59
  legal, barrister, solicitor, 65
  public relations, 62
  publishing, 64
  teaching, 57
CBI report on women and employment opportunities, 54-55, 92
child-care, 13, 39
child-care options, 39
  au pair, 45-46
  childminder, 46
  crèche, 47
  mother's help, 45
  nanny, daily, live-in, nanny share, 40-44
  nursery, day, 46
childminder, 46
Childminding Association, 46, 89
conceiving, failure to, 23
costs of childcare, 48-49
couplehood, 80

crèche, 47, 48

deciding to have a baby, 7, 9, 17
depression, post-natal, 23, 30
diabetes, 22
doctors, women and careers, 59
Down's Syndrome, 22
dual income lifestyle, 14

earnings potential and
    motherhood, 10
education, costs of, 75
employment rights and women,
    52-55
  Statutory Maternity Pay (SMP)
Equal Opportunities
    Commission, 54, 91
equal opportunities for women,
    10, 12, 54

family life, claustrophobia, 27
family structure, 12
fathers, role of, 79-83
fertility, 23
finance and having a family,
    71-77
financial independence and
    women, 11, 15
forceps and labour, 22

GIFT technique, 23
guilt and working mothers, 34

husbands, 15, 79-83
high fliers and pregnancy, 9, 24
hormonal changes in pregnancy,
    82

infertility, 22-23
lifestyle and motherhood, 7, 10
    12, 13

low paid jobs, 13

marriage, fashion and attitudes
    towards, 16
marriage, immature
    relationships, 21
marriages, second, 15
maternal instinct, 13, 17
maternity leave, 53
maternity rights, pay and
    employment, 53-55, 84,
    86-87
memorandum on equal
    opportunities in education,
    58
motherhood, ambivalent
    attitudes towards, 20
  combining with career, 9, 12,
    18
  first phase of, 35
  interruption by career, 12
  timing of, 17-28

nanny, daily, live-in, nanny
    share, 41-44
nanny, finding a, 85, 88-89
nanny share register, 44, 88
National Childbirth Trust, 88
National Nursery Examination
    Board (NNEB), 41-43
Norland Nursery Training
    College, 41
nurseries, day, 46

Older children and working
    mothers, 48
older parents, 23, 24, 30, 31, 35

parental leave, EEC government
    proposals, 56-59

pregnancy, accidental, 18
pregnancy, planning your, 25
primagravida, elderly, 20
post natal tiredness, 24
Princess Christian nannies, 41
private maternity care, 23, 74-75
public relations, career and working mothers, 62, 63
publishing, women in, 64, 65

quality time with children, 35

returning to work after pregnancy, 12, 26, 27, 33-37
role of women, report on and trends in women and employment, 12, 15, 92

setting up your own business, 26
spina bifida, 22
solicitors, women and careers, 65
Statutory Maternity Pay (SMP), 52-57, 87

stress and pregnancy, 24
support groups for working mothers, 90
support systems and childcare, 14, 40
symbol of success, baby as, 18, 19

tax reform and women, 76
test tube babies, 23

Video Baby film, 10

wife-mother stereotypes, 11
Women 2000: Mintel - report on trends, 92
  new generation of, new breed of, 14
working from home, 26
women, employment policies, 55
working in pregnancy, 24

younger mothers, 20, 30